I0416029

NUTRITION AND HEALTH

A DISTINCTION WITHOUT DIFFERENCE

Folorunsho Mejabi

NUTRITION AND HEALTH: A DISTINCTION WITHOUT DIFFERENCE

ISBN:978-1-329-68532-1

-mejabibooks@gmail.com

+234-8077837770

St. Joel Publishing

CONTENTS

NUTRITION AND HEALTH 2

INTRODUCTION 6

CHAPTER 1 8

  A-LIFESTYLE 8

CHAPTER 2 29

  B- LIFESTYLE 29

CHAPTER 3 38

  C- LIFESTYLE 38

CHAPTER 4 48

  D- LIFESTYLE 48

CHAPTER 5 54

  E- LIFESTYLE..54

CHAPTER 6 59

  F- LIFESTYLE 59

CHAPTER 7 64

  G- LIFESTYLE 64

CHAPTER 8 68

  H- LIFESTYLE 68

CHAPTER 9 72

  I- LIFESTYLE 72

CHAPTER 10 85

  J- LIFESTYLE 85

CHAPTER 11 88

   K- LIFESTYLE 88

CHAPTER 12 90

   L- LIFESTYLE 90

CHAPTER 13 93

   M- LIFESTYLE 93

CHAPTER 14 100

   N- LIFESTYLE 100

CHAPTER 15 103

   O- LIFESTYLE 103

CHAPTER 16 112

   P- LIFESTYLE 112

CHAPTER 17 118

   R- LIFESTYLE 118

CHAPTER 18 125

   S- LIFESTYLE..125

CHAPTER 19 132

   T- LIFESTYLE..132

CHAPTER 20 159

   U- LIFESTYLE 159

CHAPTER 21 161

   V- LIFESTYLE 161

CHAPTER 22 164

W- LIFESTYLE 164

CHAPTER 23 174

Y-Z- LIFESTYLE 174

INTRODUCTION

According to Thomas Edison "The doctor of the future will no longer treat the human frame with drugs, but rather will cure and prevent disease with nutrition". You hear a lot about living a healthy lifestyle, enough that the phrase 'healthy lifestyle' may be one we'd like to permanently retire. The problem is, that phrase describes the life we need to live if we want to feel good and look good.

So, what does it actually mean? Well, there are the obvious things that describe a healthy person: He or she doesn't smoke, is at a healthy weight, eats healthy foods and exercises on a regular basis. It sounds so simple; it's funny just how hard it is to do all of those things in our current world.

The good news is, you don't have to change everything at the same time. In fact, the trick to healthy living is making small changes. Take more steps each day, adding fruit to your cereal, having an extra glass of water or saying no to that second helping of buttery mashed potatoes. So, what else can you be doing to live healthy? Eating a healthy diet is another part of the healthy lifestyle. Not only can a clean diet help with weight management, it can also improve your health and quality of life as you get older. You can use this book to enhance your knowledge to determine how many calories you need and what food groups you should focus on or, if you're looking for smaller changes, you can use these tips for simple ways to change how you eat. Creating a healthy lifestyle doesn't have to mean drastic changes. In fact, drastic changes almost always lead to failure. Making small changes in how you live each day can lead to big rewards, so figure out what you can to be healthy today. Reduce the risk of heart disease, stroke and diabetes by eating not only the appropriate diets but at the right time.

Folorunsho MEJABI, M.Sc., ACA

Lagos, Nigeria

"The doctor of the future will no longer treat the human frame with drugs, but rather will cure and prevent disease with nutrition."

~Thomas Edison

CHAPTER 1

A-LIFESTYLE

- 7-Up – invented in 1920 contained Lithium – the drug commonly prescribed now to sufferers of bi-polar disorder.

- A "cork-tease" is someone who constantly talks about the wine he or she will open but never does.

- A "dumb" wine refers to the lack of odour in a wine, though it may develop a pleasing odour in the future. Many Cabernet-Sauvignons, for example, are considered "dumb." A "numb" wine, on the other hand, has no odour and no potential of developing a pleasing odour in the future.

- A 1,000-year-old popped kernel of popcorn was found in a dry cave in the south-western part of Utah.

- A 1,700-year-old funeral urn was discovered in Mexico that shows a corn god wearing a popcorn headdress.

- A 1552 B.C. Egyptian papyrus provides an early description of what seems to be diabetes and specifically mentions polyuria (frequent urination). Up until the eleventh century A.D., diabetes was typically diagnosed by "water tasters" who drank the urine of those thought to have diabetes. Those who had sweet-tasting urine were thought to have diabetes mellitus (Latin for "honey"), or Type 1 diabetes.

- A 2006 survey reveals that 6% of people in England are vegetarian, making the UK the European country with the largest proportion of its population that is vegetarian

- A 2008 study by Time Magazine approximates the number of U.S. vegetarians at 7.3 million adults or 3.2% of the population. Of these, 0.5 % or 1 million are vegans.

- A 2009 study by the Department of Human Biology, Nutrition and Toxicology Research Institute at Maastricht University in The Netherlands argues that the catechins in green tea help decrease body weight as well as maintaining body weight after weight loss.

- A 2011 study showed that women who drink two to three cups of caffeinated coffee a day were 15% less likely to develop depression over a 10-year period than those who drank one cup of coffee or less per week.

- A baby cannot taste salt until it is 4 months old. The delay may be related to the development of kidneys, which start to process sodium at about that age.

- A banana ripens quickly (overnight), when you put it into a brown paper bag with an apple or tomato.

- A Belgian named George Washington invented instant coffee in 1906 in Guatemala.

- A British study revealed that a child's IQ could help predict his or her chance for becoming a vegetarian. The higher the IQ, the more likely the child will become a vegetarian.

- A Buddhist vegetarian (su vegetarianism) will not eat any animal products nor vegetables in the Allium family such as onion, garlic, leeks, chives, and shallots because the smell of these fetid vegetables is offensive and "angers up the blood."

- A Children's Food Campaign (CFC) survey found that some baby food has as much, if not more, saturated fats and sugar as junk food.

- A Chilli's Smokehouse Bacon Triple-The-Cheese Big Mouth Burger with Jalapeno Ranch Dressing has 2,040 calories, 150 g of fat, and 4,900 mg sodium. Americans eat nearly 40 billion hamburgers a year.

- A civil penalty of up to $11,000 for each offense can be levied on any person who knowingly sells or labels as organic a product that is not produced and handled according to the National Organic Programs (NOP) regulations for organic food.

- A company in Taiwan makes dinnerware out of wheat, so you can eat your plate!

- A conventionally grown apple may be sprayed up to 16 times with over 30 different chemicals.

- A crop of newly planted grape vines takes four to five years to grow before it can be harvested.

- A cucumber is a fruit not a vegetable.

- A cup of brewed tea usually contains less than half the caffeine of a cup of coffee. It's also easy to decaffeinate loose tea at home by "rinsing" tea leaves. To rinse the leaves, begin brewing tea as usual and then remove the leaves after 20 seconds. Discard the brew and start again with fresh boiling water and the now-decaffeinated tea leaves.

- A cup of plain popcorn contains just 31 calories.

- A deficiency of calcium/vitamin D during infancy or childhood results in rickets (deformed bones). The bones can become so weak that they can't withstand the body's weight, causing bow legs or knock knees. Once malformed, bones cannot be straightened.

- A drawing from the Mayan Madrid Codex shows gods piercing their ears and sprinkling their blood over the cacao harvest, indicating a strong association between blood and cacao in Meso-American tradition.

- A durian is a large fruit with a powerful smell. Its flavour is loved by some people, but many do not like the smell.

- A durian is one of the world's biggest fruit with a strong smell

- A feminine wine is a wine that is more delicate than most. A masculine wine refers to a "big" or "full" wine.

- A few vine cuttings from the New World brought to Europe spread a tiny insect called Phylloxera vastatrix, which feeds on the roots of vines. The only way to save European grape vines was to graft native American vines to European rootstocks. Consequently, Pre-Phylloxera wine, strictly speaking, is one made in the years before Phylloxera reached the vineyards in the 1860s, though the phrase is also used to mean wine from ungrafted vines.

- A fresh bean should snap crisply and feels velvety to the touch

- A fruitarian is a type of vegetarian in which a person eats just fruits, nuts, seeds, and other plant material that can be harvested without killing the plant.

- A full seven percent of the entire Irish barley crop goes to the production of Guinness beer.

- A genetically engineered hormone called rBGH is given to cows in the U.S. to increase milk production—even though its chemical by-products may be carcinogenic. Residues of rBGH have been found in meat products, such as hamburgers sold in fast food chains.

- A half-cup of figs has as much calcium as a half-cup of milk

- A Harvard study showed that eating one serving of cooked oatmeal two to four times a week was linked to a 16% reduction in the risk of developing Type 2 diabetes. One serving five or six times a week was linked to a 39% reduction in risk.

- A hectare of conventionally farmed land produces 2½ times more potatoes than an organic one.

- A Hershey's bar was dug up after 60 years from Admiral Richard Byrd's cache at the South Pole. Having been frozen all those years, it was still edible.

- A juicer is not a blender. A blender mixes/pulverizes instead of extracts. Specifically, blenders do not separate the juice from the fibre whereas juicers or juicing machines do.

- A kernel of popcorn contains just a small amount of water. When these kernels are heated, the water turns to steam and the kernels "pop." Popcorn is different than many other grains because its shell is not water permeable, making it possible for pressure to build up until the kernel finally explodes.

- A lacto-vegetarian will eat dairy products but not eggs.

- A litre of organic milk requires 80% more land than conventional milk to produce, has 20% more global warming potential, releases 60% more nutrients into water sources, and contributes 70% more to acid rain.

- A McDonald's Big Mac has 85 mg. of cholesterol and a Wendy's Classic Double With Everything has 175 mg. of cholesterol. A single cup of ice cream has more cholesterol than 10 glazed donuts.

- A McDonald's' corn muffin has more calories than a glazed donut. A small packet of Wendy's honey mustard dressing has 280 calories.

- A normal, healthy amount of food for an average teenager or adult is about 1,800-2,600 calories a day. During a bingeing episode, it is not unusual for someone to eat 20 to 25 times that amount, which is more than 50,000 calories—which is roughly equivalent to an entire extra-large pepperoni pizza, a tub of ice cream, a package of cookies, a bag of potato chips, and an entire cake. .

- A number of researchers argue that while the human body is capable of digesting meat, our bodies are actually designed to be herbivores. For example, the human molars are similar to those of an herbivore, flat and blunt, which make them good for grinding, not gnashing and tearing.

- A person will eat an average of 35 tons of food in his or her lifetime, or 1,500 pounds of food a year.

- A person will usually swallow around 250 times during dinner.

- A person would need to walk nine miles to burn off the 923 calories found in Burger King's Double Whopper with cheese

- A pescetarian is a vegetarian who eats fish. Similar to a vegetarian diet, a pescetarian diet includes vegetables, fruits, grains, dairy, beans, and eggs. Unlike a vegetarian diet, a pescetarian diet also includes fish and shell fish. The term first originated in 1993 and is a blend of the Italian word pesce (fish) and the English word vegetarian.

- A recent study argues that people who eat tofu and other plant-based foods have a better sex life than meat-eaters It claims that certain plants influence hormone levels and sexual activity.

- A single fruit is about 125 grams on average; where ¼ of it is only water.

- A standard glass of dry red or white wine contains around 110 calories. Sweeter wine has more calories.

- A strawberry is not an actual berry, but a banana is.

- A study by North-western University found that adults who frequently attended religious activities were significantly more likely to become obese than those who didn't.

- A study reveals avocados are the world's most nutritious fruit

- A tea plant can grow into a tree that is as tall as 52 feet if its leaves are not harvested. Cultivated plants are usually pruned to waist height.

- A tomato grown in a hothouse has half the vitamin C content as a vine-ripened tomato

- A typical American eats 28 pigs in his/her lifetime.

- A typical banana travels 4,000 miles before being eaten.

- A University of Southern California study in 2009 revealed that African American girls are 50% more likely to be bulimic than white girls. Additionally, girls from families in the lowest income bracket studied are 153% more likely to be bulimic than girls from the highest income bracket.

- A watermelon contains 92% water. About six per cent of a watermelon is sugar. Many people like to eat watermelon in the summer because the fruit is cool and refreshing.

- A wine that has a musty smell, similar to wet cardboard or mold may mean that the bottle is "corked" (the bottle has a contaminated cork).

- A wine that tastes watery is said to taste "dilute." It may have been made from grapes picked during a rainstorm.

- A&W Root Beer is named after Roy Allen and Frank Wright, the founders of the company. Allen bought the recipe from a pharmacist who had perfected it for making root beer. A&W was one of the first fast food franchises.

- Aborigines and the Pima Indians of Arizona developed obesity, type 2 diabetes, and hypertension after transitioning to a Western diet.

- About 25% of all iceberg lettuce is made into fresh cut salads.

- About 60-70% of people with diabetes have mild to severe forms of nervous system damage.

- According to American Academy of Paediatrics (AAP) officials, there is currently no direct evidence proving that an organic diet leads to improved health or lower risk of disease. However, no large studies in humans have been conducted that specifically address the long-term benefits of an organic vs. conventional diet.

- According to an online survey by the Rudd Center for Food Policy and Obesity at Yale University, nearly half of the 4,000 people surveyed reported that they would give up a year of their life rather than be fat.

- According to Aztec legend, the god Quetzalcoatl brought cacao to earth but was cast out of heaven for giving it to humans. As he fled, he vowed to return one day as a "fair-skinned bearded man to save the earth."

- According to legend, coffee was discovered in the 9th century when an Ethiopian goat herder named Khaldi noticed that his normally lethargic goats were more excitable after they had nibbled the red berries from an evergreen tree. Khaldi took the berries to a Muslim holy man, who turned the raw fruit of the coffee tree into the delicious beverage.

- According to many historians, goats were the first animal to be domesticated. Goats are typically the cleanest of animals. They are much more select feeders than cows, chickens, or even dogs. They typically will not eat food that has been contaminated or that has been on the floor or ground.

- According to one study, while women view vegetarian men as more principled, they also considered them "wimps" and "less macho" than those who eat meat.

- According to the American Diabetic Association, the current means for battling obesity—such as dieting, bariatric (weight-loss) surgery, exercise—have not been able to overcome the widespread availability of low-cost, high-calorie food.

- According to the Centers for Disease Control (CDC), more than half of the adult population in the U.S. is either overweight or obese. More than one third of U.S. adults (35.7%) are obese

- According to the Centers for Disease Control and Prevention (CDC), diabetes is the sixth leading cause of death in the United States.

- According to the Dead Sea scrolls cherry seeds have satanic power

- According to the Department of Veteran Affairs, of the 7.5 million U.S. veterans who receive their health benefits from the agency, more than 70% are overweight and 20% have diabetes.

- According to the Department of Veterans Affairs, diabetes is more prevalent among military veterans than in the general population. Approximately 16% of military veterans (or about 500,000) have diabetes, compared to 6% of the general U.S. public.

- According to the U.S Census, a farm is any establishment which produces and sells, or normally would have produced or sold, $1,000 or more of agricultural products during the year. Government subsidies are included in sales.

- According to the UN, an exploding world population, intensive farming practices, and changes in climate have provided a breeding ground for an unprecedented number of merging diseases. Poultry farming, for example, may account for the global spread of bird flu. In fact, the majority of the 39 new diseases that have emerged in just one generation have come from animals, including Ebola, SARS, and the bird flu.

- Accordingly to a U.S. survey, children born to obese women are more likely to be diagnosed with autism or related developmental delays. However, researchers note that they are far from understanding what might create a link between obesity and autism.

- Additives and preservatives such as common food dyes and sodium benzoate can cause children to become more hyperactive and easily distracted than usual.

- Advantages of organic meat include reduced exposure to antibiotic-resistant bacteria.

- Adventurer and TV star Bear Grylls suffers from high levels of cholesterol, a disease that killed his father and grandfather. Bill Clinton and David Letterman also both suffer from high cholesterol.

- Advertising Age selected the McDonald's slogan "You Deserve a Break Today" as the best advertising campaign of the twentieth century. Other notable slogans were Burger King's "Burger King, Home of the Whopper" and Wendy's "Where's the Beef?"

- After Barbara Hewson from Wales was squashed by an obese person next to her on a transatlantic flight, she suffered a blood clot in her chest, torn leg muscles, and acute sciatica and was bedridden for a month. Virgin Atlantic awarded her the equivalent of US $24,100 as compensation.

- After the Boston Tea Party, tea declined in popularity in the United States. To this day, coffee remains more popular than tea.

- Agricultural efficiency has increased over the past century from 27.5 acres/worker in 1890 to 740 acres/worker in 1990.

- Alaska Natives have the highest rates of botulism in the world due to the way they butcher and store indigenous food (such as seals) under the ground in plastic bags.

- All tea is made from the leaf of the plant Camellia sinensis. The specific types of tea are made by processing the tea leaves differently.

- All wines taste like fruit. Only rarely does a wine taste like grapes—for example, Muscat or Concord wines.

- Alloxen, a byproduct of bleaching white flour which is often found in junk food, leads to diabetes in healthy experimental animals by destroying their pancreatic beta cells.

- Almonds are a member of the peach family.

- Almost 50% of organic pesticides in Europe failed to pass the European Union's safety evaluations.

- Almost 80% of food commercials aired on Saturday morning children shows are for junk food.

- Almost all lettuce is packed right in the field.

- Although anorexia is more common among young people than any other age group, it is more deadly in the elderly. From 1986 to 1990, the elderly accounted for 78% of all deaths due to anorexia.

- Although cocoa originated in Central and South America more than 4,000 years ago, now approximately 70% of the world's cacao is grown in Africa. Cote d'voire is the single largest producer of cocoa, providing roughly 40% of the world's supply.

- Although chicken is typically a low-fat meal choice, keeping the skin on the chicken or frying it turns it into a high-cholesterol food.

- Although only 2.4% of the world's crop land is planted with cotton, it accounts for 24% and 11% of the global sales of insecticide and pesticides, respectively.

- Although ready-to-drink teas and iced tea are increasing in popularity, they may not have the same polyphenol content as brewed hot tea, which has the highest polyphenol concentration.

- Although tea arrived in England in 1657, it did not immediately become popular. First sold in coffee houses, tea was heavily taxed, illegally smuggled, altered, and fought over. It took many years for it to become a quintessential English drink.

- Although yields vary from harvest to harvest, a single coffee tree usually provides only enough coffee beans in a year to fill a half-kilo (one-pound) bag of ground coffee.

- Amenorrhea occurs in anorexics because extremely low body weight can interrupt hormone functions and stop ovulation. It can permanently affect a woman's fertility.

- American businessman Charles Cretors invented large-scale commercial popcorn machines in 1893. He had the first automated machine that could pop popcorn in its own seasonings uniformly.

- American Indians are the least likely to have high cholesterol. However, white Americans and Mexican Americans are most likely to have high cholesterol.

- American Indians used to believe that spirits peacefully lived inside each popcorn kernel. When the kernels were heated, the spirits would get so angry that their "houses" would start to shake. When it got too hot, the spirits broke out of their houses in very angry burst of steam.

- Americans are the world's leading coffee consumer. They consume 450 million cups of coffee per day, or more than 150 billion cups a year.

- Americans collectively consume approximately 900 billion calories each day.

- Americans eat 2.8 billion pounds of candy each year. Nearly half of this is chocolate.

- Americans eat 20.7 pounds of candy per person annually. The Dutch eat three times as much.

- Americans eat 300–400% more fat than they should.

- Americans eat about 30 pounds of lettuce every year. That's about five times more than what we ate in the early 1900s.

- Americans eat around 17 billion quarts of popcorn every year. This amount would fill the Empire State Building 18 times.

- Americans eat more popcorn than any other country. Most of the popcorn eaten around the world is grown in the United States.

- Americans on average eat 18 acres of pizza every day.

- Americans spend 10% of their income on food, which is the lowest of any country.

- Americans spend approximately $25 billion each year on beer.

- Americans spent an estimated $267 billion dining out in 1993.

- Among the first fast food mascots was Big Boy, a plump boy with red-and-white checkered overalls with the words "Big Boy" spread across his chest. The first McDonald's mascot was "Speedee," a little chef with a hamburger hat. McDonald's later settled on the iconic Ronald McDonald—and today 96% of American children recognize him.

- An adult can starve to death within 8-12 weeks. In the final stages of starvation, adults can experience hallucinations, convulsions, severe muscle pain, and irregular heart rhythms. Organs weakened by starvation may actually burst if food is given too quickly.

- An apple is a very refreshing tonic for oily skin. It makes an excellent remedy for fine wrinkles, cracked skin, itching and inflammation

- An apple-shaped body, or excess abdominal fat, is a risk factor for Type 2 diabetes

- An average strawberry has around 200 seeds

- An avocado has more than twice as much potassium as a banana.

- An avocado is a fruit and not a vegetable! It is actually a member of the berry relatives.

- An eating disorder is characterized by abnormal eating patterns that attempt to satisfy a psychological rather than physical need. The three most common disorders are anorexia nervosa, bulimia nervosa, and binge eating disorder. Anorexia nervosa is characterized by self-starvation, weight loss, an irrational fear of gaining weight, and a distorted body image. Bulimia nervosa is characterized by a cycle of compulsive binging followed by purging through various means, such as vomiting, laxative/diuretic abuse, and extreme exercising. Binge eating disorder is the most common disorder and is characterized by frequent periods of compulsive overeating without accompanying purging behaviours.

- An estimated 16 million Americans have pre-diabetes, and many of them are unaware of their condition.

- An estimated 85% of tea that is consumed in the United States is iced tea.

- An estimated four out of five Americans start their day with a coffee.

- An etiquette writer of the 1840's advised, "Ladies may wipe their lips on the tablecloth, but not blow their noses on it."

- An Italian study argues that women who drink two glasses of wine a day have better sex than those who don't drink at all.

- An Ohio State study shows that increasing cholesterol levels can help ease autism symptoms in children.

- An orange's vitamin C content helps fight back assaults from viruses and germs, cold and fatigue.

- An ovo-lacto vegetarian diet includes both eggs and dairy products.

- An ovo-vegetarian will eat eggs but not other dairy products.

- An Oxford, England, study concluded that meat eaters were two and half times more likely to develop gallstones than non-meat eaters. Scientists concluded that the low-fat, high-fibre diet of vegetarians decreased the risk of developing gallstones.

- Ancient Mesoamerican cultures such as the Olmec, Maya, and Aztec used chocolate as medicine and as a medium in which other medicines were taken.

- Ancient Romans thought seasoning was more important than the primary flavour of wine and often added fermented fish sauce, garlic, asafoetida (onion root), lead, and absinthe.

- Annually, Americans buy nearly $2 billion in Easter candies, including 90 million chocolate Easter bunnies, 16 billion jellybeans, and 700 million marshmallow peeps.

- Anorexia affects people of all ages, genders, and ethnic backgrounds; however, young white women who are high academic achievers are more likely to develop the illness.

- Anorexia Bulimia affects up to 10% of college-aged women 13.Studies suggest that genetic factors play a significant role in the development of eating disorders. Relatives of women with anorexia are 11 times more likely to have anorexia, and relatives of women with bulimia are almost four times at greater risk for bulimia.

- Anorexia can stunt growth, cause osteoporosis, delay sexual development, cause kidney and heart problems, lower blood pressure, and cause chest and stomach pain, heartburn, constipation, and death.

- Anorexia is the third most common chronic illness in adolescents.

- Anorexia nervosa ("an"-without, "orexia"-appetite, desire) is also known as the "rich girl's syndrome."

- Anorexia nervosa (an = without, orexia = appetite), bulimia (bous = ox , limous = hunger) and binge eating disorders have been described in ancient texts, but the number of cases skyrocketed in industrialized, economically developed nations during the 1960s.

- Anorexia nervosa became an increasing problem during the Victorian era. Some researchers speculate that food was one of the few areas in life during that time where women had some control. Additionally, a woman with an appetite was associated with indulgence and lack of control. Conversely, a frail, pale, and thin woman was associated with femininity and attractiveness.

- Anorexia nervosa increased so rapidly in the 1980s in the U.S. that the disease became known as the "disorder of the 80s."

- Anorexia typically begins at or just after puberty. Bulimia occurs in slightly older females, typically around 18. More people suffer from compulsive eating disorder than from bulimia or anorexia.

- Approximately 10-15% of anorexics or bulimics are male. White males are the least likely to try to control their weight; Latino males are the most likely.

- Anthropophagites, or cannibals, are humans who eat human meat. While human flesh itself contains high-quality protein, cannibalism in most cultures likely served a more symbolic than nutritional purpose.

- Apples float in water because they are 25% air.

- Apples, not caffeine, are more efficient at waking you up in the morning.

- Apples, potatoes, and onions all taste the same when eaten with your nose plugged.

- Approximately 11% of adult Americans of Asian descents are considered obese compared to the nation's average, which is 35%. However, diseases associated with obesity can start at lower BMIs for them.

- Approximately 11% of all Americans aged 65-74 have diabetes. About 20% of those over 75 years old have diabetes, and nearly half of them are unaware they have the disease.

- Approximately 17 million U.S. residents have been diagnosed with diabetes, which is nearly 10% of the estimated 170 million people suffering from diabetes worldwide.

- Approximately 25 gallons of water are needed to produce 1 pound of wheat. Around 2,500 gallons of water are needed to produce 1 pound of meat. Many vegetarians argue that more people eating a meat-free diet would lower the strain that meat production puts on the environment.

- Approximately 30–50% of children born in 2000 will develop type 2 diabetes mellitus, a leading cause of preventable blindness, kidney failure, heart disease, stroke, and amputations.

- Approximately 40% of all meals eaten each day in the US are eaten outside of the home.

- Approximately 40% of almonds produced in the world are made for chocolate products.

- Approximately 60% of the farmers in the United States are 55 years old or older. Aging farmers have led to concern about the long-term health of family farms.

- Approximately 70% of popcorn sold in America is eaten in the home. The other 30% is eaten in theatres, stadiums, school, etc.

- Approximately 70% of the nearly $500 million spent on candy during the week leading up to Easter is for chocolate.

- Approximately 71 million pounds of chocolate candy is sold during the week leading up to Easter. Only 48 million pounds of chocolate is sold during Valentine's week. In contrast, over 90 million pounds of chocolate candy is sold in the last week of October leading up to Halloween.

- Approximately 97% of U.S. farms are operated by families, family partnerships, or family corporations.

- Arabs were the first to cultivate coffee trees on the Arabian Peninsula. Arabs typically roasted and boiled coffee, or qahwa, which is Arabic for "the wine of Islam."

- Archaeologists found grape pips (seeds), usually considered evidence of winemaking, dating from 8000 B.C. in Turkey, Syria, Lebanon, and Jordan. The oldest pips of cultivated vines were found in (then Soviet) Georgia from 7000-5000 B.C.

- As an easy way to reduce grains in your diet, spread peanut butter on celery rather than bread.

- As of 2006, there were more people in the world who are overweight than malnourished.

- Asparagus is a good source of vitamins A, C and E, B-complex vitamins, potassium and zinc

- Asparagus is high in glutathione, an important anti-carcinogen

- At least 2.8 million people die each year as a result of being overweight or obese. Although once associated with high-income countries, obesity is also becoming prevalent in low- and middle-income countries.

- At one time in the late 18th century, tea in Britain was predominantly imported through illegal methods. Smugglers would often mix tea (most often green tea) with other types of leaves and additives to increase their profits. Often these additives were poisonous. The British government intervened in 1785 and lowered taxes, which made tea more affordable and wiped out illegal smuggling activity.

- At some fast food chains, both in U.S. and in other countries, managers are rewarded bonuses when they reduce employee wages to save money.

- At the centre of Greek social and intellectual life was the symposium, which literally means, "drinking together." Indeed, the symposium reflects Greek fondness for mixing wine and intellectual discussion.

- At what stage of life a person becomes obese can affect his or her ability to lose weight. In childhood and puberty, excess calories are converted into new fat cells (hyperplastic obesity), while excess calories consumed in adulthood only serve to expand existing fat cells (hypertrophic obesity).

- Aunt Jemima pancake flour, invented in 1889, was the first ready-mix food to be sold commercially.

- Autumn is the peak time for popcorn consumption, followed by the winter months. Popcorn sales taper off during the spring and summer.

- Avocado has more fat content than any other fruit.

- Avocado leaves are harmful to animals and the fruits may also poisonous to some birds

- Avocados are rich in monounsaturated fat, which is easily burned for energy.

- avocados are the world's most nutritious fruit.

"The greatest wealth is Health."

~Unknown

CHAPTER 2

B- LIFESTYLE

- Babaco is gorgeous torpedo shaped fruit. It's also named as champagne fruit since it has a fizzy flesh.

- Banana is not a fruit in reality, it is a herb

- Banana ripens quickly in brown paper bag

- Banana slip accidents in Britain

- Banana trees are not actually trees – they are giant herbs.

- Banana's are most likely the first fruit ever to be grown on a farm.

- Banana-a cure for heartburn

- Bananas are a great source of potassium. Potassium helps build muscle power and keeps your body fluids in balance.

- Bananas are about 99.5% fat free.

- Bananas are allergic for some people. These allergies are oral and latex.

- Bananas are easily digestible

- Bananas are high in sugar,

- Bananas are the number one fruit crop in the world. They are the 4th largest overall crop, after wheat, rice, and corn. They grow in more than 100 countries on farms. India grows more bananas than any other country. The Philippines, China, and Ecuador are the next three top producers of bananas.

- Bananas have a natural antacid effect in the body, so if you suffer from heartburn, try eating a banana for soothing relief.

- Because bananas are easy to digest and are very nutritious they are the first fruit offered to babies.

- Because carrots greens, rhubarb greens, or the peels of oranges and grapefruit contain toxic substances, these greens and skins should not be juiced. However, the pithy white part of citrus just underneath the skin is very nutritious. To benefit from this pith, grate the peel off oranges and grapefruits instead of peeling.

- Because cholesterol is oil based and blood is water based, if cholesterol were just dumped into a person's bloodstream, it would congeal into unusable globs. The body has to package it in miniscule protein particles called lipoproteins.

- Because enzyme degradation occurs almost immediately after juicing, most experts do not recommend storing homemade juice longer than 24 hours.

- Because grapes in the Southern Hemisphere are picked during what is spring in the Northern Hemisphere, a 1999 Australian wine could be six months older than a 1999.

- Because homemade raw juice is not pasteurized, it is important to wash fruit and veggies thoroughly (even organic ones) and to drink raw juice immediately after it is made to minimize the risk of food-borne illness, such as hepatitis. Additionally, the antioxidants and other phytonutrients start to break down almost immediately once they are exposed to light and air.

- Because it is illegal to hunt alligators in the U.S., alligator meat must be purchased from farms. Once an alligator is 5 to 7 feet long, it is ready to be slaughtered for meat, hide, and teeth.

- Because juicing removes fibre from food—and fibre is an essential part of healthful diet and long-term health—dieticians don't recommend replacing regular meals with juices except for short-term weight loss or cleansing programs.

- Because juicing removes fibre from fruit and veggies, the body absorbs fructose sugar from fruit juice more easily, which can upset blood sugar levels. Because of this, many health professional encourage people to drink more veggie juices and to limit fruit juice to a glass a day.

- Because McDonald's initially did not want its customers to stay and socialize, they prohibited newspaper boxes, candy machines, telephones, pinball machines, jukeboxes, and other types of entertainment. They also installed uncomfortable chairs to deter customers from lingering.

- Because sugar was strictly rationed during WWII, candy was not plentiful. Consequently, Americans ate three times as much popcorn during this time as usual.

- Because tea absorbs moisture, it is important to store loose tea or tea bags in a tin or sealed jar.

- Because the organs and systems in a foetus are not able to metabolize and excrete caffeine fully, caffeine can stay in its blood 10 times longer than in an adult. Because of this, physicians advise that pregnant women drink a moderate (less than 200 milligrams) amount coffee per day.

- Bees contribute to more than $15 billion worth of crops every year through pollination.

- Beet greens contain notable amounts of calcium, iron, magnesium and phosphorus

- Beet greens, parsley, spinach, and watercress yield very rich and thick juices. They are very strong flavoured and taste best when combined with other fruits and vegetables. For example, green vegetable juice mixed with carrot juice procures a sweeter vegetable flavour.

- Beet roots are high in carbohydrate levels and should therefore be used sparingly

- Before menopause, women typically have lower total cholesterol levels than men. However, after menopause, their LDL levels tend to rise. Scientists believe that oestrogen helps keep cholesterol levels down.

- Before the discovery of insulin in 1921, physicians would often put their patients on starvation or semi-starvation diets, recommending they eat only foods such as oatmeal.

- Benjamin Franklin was an early American vegetarian (though he later became a meat-eater again). He introduced tofu to America in 1770.

- Besides Americans, the two other largest drinkers of coffee are the French and the Germans. These three countries drink approximately 65% of the total coffee consumed in the world.

- Besides churches and monasteries, two other great medieval institutions derived much of their income from wine: hospitals and universities. The most famous medieval wine-endowed hospital (now a museum) is the beautiful Hôtel-Dieu in Beaune, France.

- Bilberries are supposed to help improve night-time vision.

- Bilberry contains nutrients that are good for eyes.

- Bilimbi fruit is similar to star fruit. The tree of Bilimbi is more cold-sensitive than the carambola tree. The fruit is more effective for several human ailments.

- Bizarre popcorn flavours include Beer-flavoured Pub-Corn, Yo-Pop's Butterfinger Crunch Popcorn, KukuRuZa's Buffalo Blue Cheese Popcorn, Popcorn Palace's Jalapeno popcorn, Jolly Time's Mallow Magic Yummy Marshmallow Flavour Microwave Popcorn, Popcorn Pavilion's Brown Butter & Sea Salt Popcorn, Kernel Encore's Pumpkin popcorn, Popcorn polis' Cupcake popcorn, and 479° Popcorn's Black Truffle and White Cheddar popcorn.

- Black currant juice can be used to soothe sore throats and colds

- Black tea is the world's most popular type of tea .Black tea constitutes around 75% of the world's tea consumption.

- Black tea is called "red tea" in China.

- Black tea is the most common tea beverage in the United States, the U.K., and Europe. Green tea is popular in Japan and China. Oolong and white tea are in general less popular.

- Black tea undergoes the longest process of oxidation. White tea undergoes the shortest.

- Blackberry juice was used to dye cloth navy blue and indigo

- Blacks have the highest obesity rates (47.8%), followed by Hispanics (42.5%) and whites (32.6%). Asians have the lowest obesity rates (10.8%).

- Blue and purple fruits help your memory.

- Boodles jewellers made a handcrafted diamond teabag worth $15,250. As the most expensive teabag in the world, it contains 280 diamonds and is being used to raise money for a children's charity in Manchester, England.

- Both the American Dietetic Association and the American Diabetes Association say that popcorn can be exchanged for bread for people on weight control diets.

- Both the leaves and seeds aid digestion, relieve intestinal gas, pain and distension

- Bovine Spongiform Encephalopathy (BSE) or Mad Cow Disease cannot be killed in meat by cooking. The interval between the virus getting into the body and the final illness is about one to two years in small animals to an estimated five to 30 years in humans.

- Brains are unhealthy to eat because they are high in cholesterol and fat. For example, a single serving of a 140 g. can of "pork brains in milk gravy" contains 3,500 mg. of cholesterol, 1170% of the USRDA.

- Britain is the second-largest nation of tea drinkers per capita. Ireland is the first.

- British physician Sir Richard Morton (1637-1698) is considered to have recorded the earliest medical description of anorexic illness. He reported two cases, one in which the girl was "sad and anxious" and "pored over books." The second case was a boy who was "prone to studying too hard."

- Broccoli contains twice the vitamin C of an orange

- Broccoli is a modest source of vitamin A and alpha-tocopherol vitamin E

- Broccoli is a vegetable with a nervous system. Primitive though it may be, it CAN feel pain.

- Bubbles in wine have been observed since ancient Greece and were attributed to the phases of the moon or to evil spirits.

- Bulimia ("bous"-ox, "limous"-hunger) nervosa first entered the English language in the late 1970s, though descriptions of bulimic behaviour have been found in ancient texts.

- Bulimics Approximately 50% of anorexics also develop bulimia. Bulimics almost always binge on "forbidden food," such as junk food or fast food. They often feel powerless to stop eating during binges.

- Bulimics who use laxatives believe they can prevent their bodies from absorbing food by fast elimination. However, nutrients are absorbed in the small intestine, and laxatives work mainly in the large bowel. The only weight a person "loses" with a laxative is water. Bulimics often overuse laxatives, which can lead to inflammation of the intestinal lining, damage to the colon, severe dehydration, and decreased levels of potassium and sodium. Ironically, overuse of laxatives can also cause constipation.

- Burger King's Double Whopper with cheese contains 923 calories. A man would need to walk for about nine miles to burn it off. Adding French fries and a large cola brings the total calories to an amazing 1,500 calories (2/3 of an adult man's recommended daily caloric intake).

- Burger King's Triple Whopper with cheese has an amazing 1,230 calories. Hardies Monster Thick burger has 1,420 calories and 2,770 grams of sodium. Carl's Jr.'s Double Six hamburger has 1,520 calories and 111 grams of fat. Most people need only 44-66 grams of fat per day, and most of them should come from sources like nuts, fish, and olive oil.

- By eating a whole apple, you can get up to 15 times the amount of fibre of drinking juiced apples.

- By the end of the twentieth century, one out of eight American workers had at some time been employed by McDonald's and 96% of Americans had visited McDonald's at least once. It was also serving an estimated 22 million Americans every day and even more abroad.

- By volume, popcorn is America's favourite snack food.

"Physical fitness is not only one of the most important keys to a healthy body; it is the basis of dynamic and creative intellectual activity."

~John F. Kennedy

CHAPTER 3

C- LIFESTYLE

- Cocoa trees can live to be 200 years old, but they produce marketable cocoa beans for only 25 years.

- Caffeine is the most commonly used drug in the world, and high doses can have serious health effects, including muscle weakness, heart irregularities, and infertility Children and teenagers consume more than 64 gallons of soft drinks per year.

- Caffeine: there are 100 to 150 milligrams of caffeine in an eight-ounce cup of brewed coffee, 10 milligrams in a six-ounce cup of cocoa, 5 to 10 milligrams in one ounce of bittersweet chocolate, and 5 milligrams in one ounce of milk chocolate.

- California is the fourth-largest wine producer in the world, after France, Italy, and Spain.

- California, New York, and Florida lead the United States in wine consumption.

- California's Frank Epperson invented the Popsicle in 1905 when he was 11-years-old.

- Capsaicin, which makes hot peppers "hot" to the human mouth, is best neutralized by casein, the main protein found in milk.

- Carl Karcher of Anaheim, California, launched Carl's Jr in 1956. They were mini versions of the restaurant he already owned and, hence, he called them Carl's Jr.

- Carrots have zero fat content.

- Cast iron skillets used to be the leading source of iron in the American diet!

- Celebrities who have had a history of eating disorders include Paula Abdul, Karen Carpenter, Jane Fonda, Elton John, Princess Diana, Lynn Redgrave, Billy Bob Thornton, and Joan Rivers.

- Celery is the best vegetable source of naturally occurring sodium.

- Certain diseases—such as cystic fibrosis, pancreatitis, hemochromatosis, and Cushing's syndrome—may cause pancreatic beta cell destruction that leads to diabetes.

- Certain professions such as dancing, modelling, and horse racing have higher-than-average rates of eating disorders.

- Champagne, one of the world's greatest sparkling wines, is popularly but erroneously thought to have been invented by the Benedictine monk Dom Pierre Perignon (1638-1715). Although he did not invent or discover champagne, he founded many principles and processes in its production that are still in use today. And he purportedly declared upon drinking the bubbly beverage, "I am drinking stars."

- Chempedak fruit is really not too big. It just has the shape of long water melon but the whole fruit is only about 3 Kg.

- Cherimoya seeds are poisonous, and ought to not be eaten, like the skin.

- Cherry seeds believed to have satanic power

- Chewing gum while peeling onions will keep you from crying!

- Chewing juice helps the digestive process

- Chicken today contains 266 percent more fat than it did 40 years ago.

- Chicory contains inulin, which helps diabetics regulate their blood sugar levels

- Chicory is beneficial for digestion, the circulatory system and the blood

- Chicory is closely related to lettuce and dandelion but is a member of the sunflower family

- Chicory leaves are a good source of calcium, vitamin A and potassium

- Children who eat organic foods have lower levels of pesticides in their urine

- Child safety seat manufacturers have begun to make bigger models after a recent study showed that over 250,000 U.S. children age 6 and under are too fat to use the standard models.

- Childhood obesity affects self-esteem, which can affect employment and higher education later in life. In addition to a social stigma, childhood obesity has serious health consequences.

- Childhood trauma has been associated with a greater risk of becoming overweight or obese for both boys as for girls. The risk was even higher for kids whose mothers were obese, because obese parents may contribute to family health problems, which lead to traumatic life events.

- Children with working mothers have a greater risk of becoming obese, even if they have a full-time stay-at-home father

- China is the world's largest producer of tea. In 2009, China produced 1,359,000 tonnes; India was second with 979,000 tonnes.

- China's Beijing Duck Restaurant can seat 9,000 people at one time.

- Chinese cabbage has anti-inflammatory properties

- Chinese cabbage is low in calories and low in sodium

- Chocolate beans Over 3.8 million tons of cocoa beans are produced each year .

- Chocolate has evolved into such a massive industry that between 40 and 50 million people depend on cocoa for their livelihood.

- Chocolate became one of the earliest American exports when, in the early sixteenth century, both Columbus and Cortez brought cocoa beans back to Spain.

- Chocolate can kill dogs; it directly affects their heart and nervous system.

- Chocolate contains phenyl ethylamine (PEA), a natural substance that is reputed to stimulate the same reaction in the body as falling in love.

- Chocolate has traditionally been associated with magical, medicinal, and mythical properties. In fact, in Latin, cacao trees are called Theobroma Cacao, or "food of the gods."

- Chocolate is so important to cacao farmers in Indonesia that they built a 20-foot statue of a pair of hands simply holding a cacao pod.

- Chocolate melting in a person's mouth can cause a more intense and longer-lasting "buzz" than kissing.

- Chocolate melts because it contains cocoa butter, the fat extracted from cocoa beans

- Chocolate was included in WWII soldier rations. According to army specification, it was designed to taste just "a little better than a boiled potato" so soldiers would not eat it too quickly.

- Dark chocolate compliments red wine .Champagne and sparkling wine are too acidic to go well with dark chocolate. Red wine typically compliments it the best.

- Cholesterol is a type of lipid (fat) that is essential for all animal life—in the right amounts. It performs three essential functions: 1) Helps make the outer coating of cells, 2) Makes up the bile acids that work to digest food in the intestine, and 3) Allows the body to make Vitamin D and hormones, such as testosterone in men and oestrogen in women.

- Cholesterol is important for an embryo's healthy development. Nearly 1 in 9,000 babies is born with a birth defect linked to the foetus' failure to make the cholesterol it needs.

- Cholesterol is produced in the liver or intestines. A human liver produces about 1 g. of cholesterol per day.

- Cholesterol protects the integrity of cell membranes and keeps cells healthy and strong. If a person's cholesterol level were 0 (an impossibility), his cell membranes would be dry and cracked and all the cell content would leak out.

- Cigarette Smoking increases levels of "bad" cholesterol

- Cilantro is a member of the carrot family

- Cilantro may be useful to treat urinary tract infections

- Clementines are popular in the winter months.

- Clinical research found that babies who breastfeed at least three months had a lower incidence of Type 1 diabetes and may be less likely to become obese as adults.

- Coca Cola was originally green.

- Coca-Cola originally included coca derivatives such as cocaine in their sodas, which at the time was not illegal. It was originally served as a "brain tonic and intellectual soda fountain beverage."

- Cockroach repellent fruit

- Coconut water can be used in an emergency as a substitute for blood plasma.

- Coffee contains antioxidants, which helps prevent free radicals from damaging cells. One study found that a typical servicing (approximately 9 oz) of coffee contains more antioxidants than a serving of grape juice, blueberries, raspberries, or oranges.

- Coffee filter Metal filters can create more flavour but also more sediment .The health effects of coffee depend largely on how coffee is prepared. For example, coffee paper filters remove oily components called diterpenes, which have been linked to coronary heart disease. Metal filters, however, do not remove these oily components.

- Coffee is the world's most recognizable smell.

- Coffee trees are cultivated in over 70 countries, mostly in Africa, South Asia, Southeast Asia, and Latin America.

- Coffee was banned three times in three different cultures: once in Mecca in the 16th century, once when Charles II in Europe banned the drink in an attempt to quiet an on-going revolution, and once when Frederick the Great banned coffee in Germany in 1677 because he was concerned people were spending too much money on the drink.

- Coffee was imported from Arabia to Europe through Venice in the 1600s. While some monks urged Pope Clemente VIII to outlaw the "Muslim" drink, the pope argued that the drink was so good that it would be a "sin" to let only "pagans drink it." Coffee thus began to spread across Europe.

- Coffee was originally regarded as a wonder drug in Yemen and Arabia and was taken only at the advice of a doctor. Many saw coffee as a brain tonic or as a way to stimulate religious visions.

- Columbus's son Ferdinand recorded that when the Mayans dropped some cacao beans, "they all stopped to pick it up, as though an eye had fallen." Columbus, who was searching for a route to India, did not see the potential of the cacao market and mistook them for shrivelled almonds.

- Commercial chocolate usually contains such low amounts of cacao solids that it is more likely the sugar that chocolate lovers are addicted to.

- Common diseases that are caused by nutritional deficiencies include beriberi (Vitamin B1-thiamine), pellagra (B3-niacin), anaemia (B12-cobalamin), and scurvy (C-ascorbic acid).

- Compulsive (or binge) eating disorder is similar to bulimia in several ways. In both disorders, a person feels guilt and remorse about overeating. However, people who suffer from compulsive eating disorder do not purge. They also are often overweight or obese, placing them at a higher risk for developing cardiovascular disease and high blood pressure.

- Contrary to popular belief, popcorn is not the only corn able to pop. Many flint and dent corns also pop, but their flakes are smaller. Additionally, some varieties of rice, milo, millet, and sorghum also pop. Some varieties of quinoa, a sacred Incan food, also pops like popcorn, as does amaranth.

- Contrary to traditional belief, smelling the cork reveals little about the wine. Instead, if a server or sommelier hands you a cork, you should look for the date and other identifying information (inexpensive wine won't have these features). Additionally, look for mold, drying, cracking, or breaks in the cork.

- Conventional chicken and pork are 33% more likely to contain bacteria resistant to three or more antibiotics than organic poultry or pork are.

- Conventionally grown apples have more pesticide residue than any other fruit or vegetable

- Conventionally grown apples, celery, sweet bell peppers, peaches, strawberries, imported nectarines, grapes, spinach, lettuce, cucumbers, domestic blueberries, potatoes, green beans, kale, and other greens are among the fruits and vegetables with the highest levels of pesticides.

- Conventionally grown onions, sweet corn, pineapples, avocado, cabbage, sweet peas, asparagus, mangos, eggplant, kiwi, domestic cantaloupe, sweet potatoes, grapefruit, watermelon, and mushrooms have some of the lowest pesticide levels.

- Conversation hearts" started in the 1860s, and currently the New England Confectionery Company (NECCO) produces about 8 billion Sweethearts per year, all within the six weeks before Valentine's Day.

- Corn dextrin, a common thickener used in junk food, is also the glue on envelopes and postage stamps.

- Cracker Jack originated in Chicago and was the first to use toys to target junk food to children.

- Cranberries are sorted for ripeness by bouncing them; a fully ripened cranberry can be dribbled like a basketball.

- Cream does not weigh as much as milk.

- Critics of fast food argue that it advocates a pernicious consumerism that destroys both the environment and health of the world. Some critics warn of "the McDonaldization of America" in which fast food chains threaten small businesses and homogenize American life.

- Cupuacu pulp is also used in cosmetics products such as body lotions, as it is highly hydrating, similar to cocoa butter.

- Currant juice can be used to soothe sore throats and colds.

- Currently, 800 million people suffer from hunger and malnutrition worldwide. Around 16 million will die from it. If conventional farming were replaced by organic farming, the number of people suffering would explode to 1.3 billion, assuming farmers use the same amount of land they are using now.

- Apple seeds contain cyanide and should be removed before juicing

- Cyrus McCormick is considered the "Father of Modern Agriculture." He invented the world's first mechanical reaper in 1831, which helped replace manpower for machine power to harvest crops. His invention is often cited as key in the westward expansion of the United States. Jo Anderson, a slave, also worked with McCormick to develop the mechanical reaper.

"An apple a day keeps the doctor away"

~Proverb

CHAPTER 4

D- LIFESTYLE

- Daily candy and junk food intake in children has been linked to violence later in life, though experts are not sure if it is the candy itself or the way it is given to children that creates the association.

- Damage to the foetus's brain either during pregnancy or during birth has been shown to contribute to ADHD and other personality traits associated with eating disorders.

- Damson fruit is more effective to create fruit paste or cheese. It's perfectly made for Christmas treat.

- Dandelion greens are high in vitamin A in the form of antioxidant carotenoid and vitamin C

- Dandelion is beneficial to digestion and is an antiviral that may be useful in the treatment of AIDS and herpes

- Dandelion root contains inulin, which lowers blood sugar in diabetics

- Dangerous fast food ingredients that have been linked to various cancers and/or obesity includes MSG, trans fat, sodium nitrite, BHA, BHT, propyl gallate, aspartame, Acesulfame-K, Olestra, potassium bromate, and food colouring Blue 1 and 2, Red 3, Green 3, and Yellow 6.

- Dark chocolate has been shown to be beneficial to human health, but milk chocolate, white chocolate, and other varieties are not. For dark chocolate to be beneficial, cacao or chocolate liquor should be the first ingredient listed, not sugar.

- Dark green vegetables include more vitamin C than light green colour vegetables

- Darker Green lettuce leaves are more nutritious than lighter green leaves.

- Darker shades of wine (the deepest, blackest reds and the most golden whites) usually come from warm climates and are rich and ripe. Lighter colours, especially in white wines, come from cooler climates and are lighter and less lush.

- DEFRA (Department for Environment, Food, and Rural Affairs) estimates that organic tomato production in the UK releases almost three times the nutrient pollution and uses 25% more water per kg of fruit than normal production.

- Delicious oranges in the world are grown in Florida

- Dennis Quaid battled anorexia after shedding weight to play a man dying from tuberculosis in the film Wyatt Earp in the mid-1990s.

- Depression, loneliness, poor self-esteem, substance abuse, feelings of inadequacy, anger, and anxiety are common among people who develop eating disorders. Additionally, those who are praised or ridiculed for their weight or sexual development are also at greater risk.

- Despite some past research suggesting a link between C-sections and obesity, more recent research argues that babies born by caesarean deliveries are no more likely to be obese in life than babies born vaginally.

- Diabetes in the United States alone costs $200 billion annually. This figure includes direct medical costs, such as insulin, amputations, and hospitalizations as well as indirect costs, such as lost productivity, early retirement, and disability.

- Diabetes insipidus (water diabetes) is a condition completely different from diabetes mellitus. Diabetes insipidus is characterized by a problem with the kidneys in which the kidneys are unable to concentrate urine adequately due to a deficiency in the antidiuretic hormone (ADH).

- Diabetes is responsible for over one million amputations each year, a large percentage of cataracts, and at least 5% of blindness worldwide.

- Diabetes is the leading cause of kidney failure, accounting for 44% of new cases in 2005.

- Diabetes is the main cause of blindness in individuals aged 20-74 in the United States. Experts emphasize that early detection and treatment could prevent up to 90% of cases of blindness that are related to diabetes.

- Diabetes mellitus is a general name that encompasses several types of diabetes, including Type 1, Type 2, gestational, and variations such as maturity-onset diabetes in the young (MODY) and latent autoimmune diabetes of adulthood (LADA). What they all have in common is the inability to self-regulate levels of blood glucose (cellular fuel) in the body.

- Diabetics have a higher risk of gingivitis than non-diabetics, which may lead to bone and tooth loss. However, only about half of Hispanics with diabetes regularly visit a dentist compared to 58% of African-Americans and 70% of non-Hispanic whites with diabetes.

- Did you know? George Washington Carver was largely responsible for popularizing the peanut as a food in America.

- Dirty cantaloupes can spread bacteria. In 2011, 21 people died in the United States from cantaloupes having listeria bacteria.

- Don't eat bananas on an empty stomach; combining them with a bit of protein will help to normalize the insulin response caused by the sugar in the banana.

- Doughnuts most likely originated in Germany and were brought to New York by Dutch settlers who called them olykoeks (oily cakes). The hole in the centre was developed by the Pennsylvania Dutch perhaps because the shape provided easier dunking in coffee or made it easier to fry the donuts more thoroughly. Dunkin Donuts sells 6.4 million donuts per day (2.3 billion per year).

- Dried fruits contain more calories than fresh fruits. Since drying process takes out water and volume

- Drinking a 12 oz. can of soda is akin to eating 14 teaspoons of sugar. Drinking one can of soda a day can cause a person to gain 15 pounds in one year.

- Drinking moderate amounts of wine may lead to more enjoyable sex for women

- Due to anti-German sentiment during WWI, an alternative name for a hamburger (which was derived from the Hamburg steak sandwiches eaten on immigrant ships between Hamburg, Germany, and America in the 1800s) was "salisbury steak." It was named after Dr. Salisbury who prescribed ground beef for patients suffering from anaemia, asthma, and other illnesses.

- Due to childhood obesity, depression, diabetes, asthma, gallstones, orthopaedic diseases, and other obesity-related conditions are all on the rise in children.

- Due to repeated vomiting, bulimics may develop painful cracks in the corners of their mouths called cheilosis.

- Durian is one of the world's biggest fruit

- During an average person's life, they will consume about 60,000 pounds of food.

- During Saturday morning cartoons, children see an average of 8 junk food ads per 10 minutes of cartoons in the United States.

- During the 1930s, extruded snacks were invented by an animal feed technician, Edward Wilson, whose Korn Kurls, an early precursor to Cheetos, became popular after WWII.

- During the early 1900s, the hamburger was thought to be polluted, unsafe to eat, and food for the poor. Street carts, not restaurants, typically served them.

- During the Middle Ages, fasting was believed to bring a person closer to God. In the 1300s, for example, St. Catherine of Siena was famous for her ability to live on very small amounts of food. Supposedly, she also would make herself vomit by sticking a twig down her throat.

- During WWII, American soldiers were known as G.I. Joes. Because they drank large amounts of coffee, the drink soon earned the popular nickname "a cup of Joe."

- During WWII, the Germans designed an exploding, chocolate-covered, thin steel bomb designed to blow up seven seconds after a piece was broken off.

"The only way to keep your health is to eat what you don't want, drink what you don't like, and do what you'd rather not."

~Mark Twain

CHAPTER 5

E- LIFESTYLE

- Each ½ cup of fruit has about 60 calories, so 4–5 cups of juiced fruit has the equivalent of about 480–600 calories in each serving. In other words, portions still matter even when juicing. Juice can contain more calories than some sodas.

- Each American eats an average of 51 pounds of chocolate per year.

- Each cocoa tree can produce approximately 2,500 beans. It takes a cacao tree four to five years to produce its first beans.

- Early Roman women were forbidden to drink wine, and a husband who found his wife drinking was at liberty to kill her. Divorce on the same grounds was last recorded in Rome in 194 B.C.

- Eating 6 large carrots is equivalent to drinking 8 ounces of carrot juice.

- Eating an apple is a more reliable method of staying awake than consuming a cup of coffee. The natural sugar in an apple is more potent than the caffeine in coffee.

- Eating disorders are associated with unstable or troubled family relationships. However, even loving and nurturing families may inadvertently foster an eating disorder by overemphasizing thinness or by having overly high expectations.

- Eating disorders include anorexia nervosa, bulimia nervosa, and eating disorders not otherwise specified (EDNOS), under which binge eating disorder falls.

- Eating disorders usually begin in males around age 12–14; however, boys as young as 6 years old have been diagnosed. Eating disorders in boys usually begin for different reasons from girls. For example, nonathletic boys are less likely to develop an eating disorder than those who participate in sports. Nonathletic girls run the same risk as athletic girls.

- Eating fast food can result in high levels of insulin, which has been linked to rising incidences of Type 2 Diabetes. In fact, more than 600,000 new cases of diabetes are diagnosed each year.

- Eating fresh figs during pregnancy helps from prolonged labour and weakness after childbirth

- Eating fruits avoids miscarriage

- Eating fruits reduce the risk of diseases

- Eating grapefruit protect from diabetes

- Eating junk food while pregnant or breast feeding raises the risk of producing obese children

- Eating lemons make you live longer.

- Eating more fruits and vegetables could significantly reduce the risk of many chronic diseases, high B.P, obesity, heart disease and some cancers.

- Eating one meal of fish a week reduces your chances of getting a heart attack by 50%.

- EGG:One large egg contains 185 milligrams of cholesterol

- Eggplants are actually fruits, and classified botanically as berries.

- Eggs are a good source of protein

- Eggs contain most of the recognised vitamins with the exception of vitamin C.

- Eggs contain the highest quality food protein known. All parts of an egg are edible, including the shell which has high calcium content.

- Eggs labelled as organic must come from organically reared chickens. To be an organically reared chicken, the bird has to eat 80% organic food for 6 weeks prior to laying its egg. Organic eggs and chickens should not be confused with free-range chickens, which can roam freely and eat whatever they like. To conform to the organic requirements, an organic chicken is allowed 1 square meter of space per 25 pounds of chicken. A chicken can be both organic and free-range.

- Eli Whitney's (1765—1825) invention of the cotton gin catapulted the rise of cotton production in the Deep South which, some historians note, led to an increase in slavery and contributed to slavery issues.

- Endo-cannabinoids, the chemical that triggers the "munchies," is akin to the active chemical cannabinoids in marijuana. There are endocannabinoid (EC) receptors all over the body, including the brain, gastrointestinal tract, and fat cells. An overactive EC system can lead to obesity.

- Oenologists are wine chemists who analyse samples of wine and advise winemakers

- Eskimo ice cream is neither icy, nor creamy!

- Ethical vegans are vegans who reject the commodity status of animals or animals that are used for shelter, food, or clothing.

- European wines are named after their geographic locations (e.g., Chassagne-Montrachet Morgeot and Bordeaux) while non-European wines (e.g., Pinot Noir and Merlot) are named after different grape varieties.

- Even "metabolically healthy" obese people are at higher risk for diabetes and heart disease.

- Even fat-free food can be rich in sugar. In many cases, manufactures will replace fat calories with sugar calories so the food remains desirable to the palate.

- Even small changes in household routines can reduce obesity risk in kids, such as restricting TV time and increasing sleep time.

- Every 10 seconds someone dies from diabetes-related causes globally. Every year nearly 3.5 million people in the world die due to diabetes. The death rate is expected to rise by 25% over the next decade.

- Every month, approximately nine out of 10 American children visit a McDonald's restaurant.

- Every time you lick a stamp, you're consuming 1/10 of a calorie.

- Evidence in Peru suggests that popcorn existed as early as 4700 B.C., making it one of the oldest forms of corn. Peruvians didn't just pop their corn; they also ground it into flour to cook in other ways.

- Experts report that diabetes decreases life expectancy by five to 10 years.

"To insure good health: eat lightly, breathe deeply, live moderately, cultivate cheerfulness, and maintain an interest in life."

~William Londen

CHAPTER 6

F- LIFESTYLE

- Famous songs about tea are "Tea for Two," "No, No, Nanette," and "When I Take My Sugar to Tea."

- Famous vegetarians include Leonardo da Vinci, Henry Ford, Brad Pitt, Albert Einstein, Ozzy Osborne, and (debatably) Hitler.

- Farm and ranch families comprise just 2% of the U.S. population.

- Farmers have cleared more than 35% of Earth's ice-free land surface for agriculture. This is an area that is 60 times larger than the combined area of all the world's cities and suburbs. Until organic farming can produce crops competitive with conventional methods, it cannot be considered a viable option for the majority of the world.

- Farmers often plant tall, dense trees on the edges of fruit farms. These trees provide a windbreak, which helps prevent soil erosion.

- Farmers today produce 262% more food with 2% fewer inputs (such as seeds, labour, fertilizers) than they did in 1950.

- Farming began around 10,000 B.C. during the First Agricultural Revolution, when nomadic tribes began to farm. Additionally, this is when the eight so-called "founder crops" of agriculture appeared: 1) emmer wheat, 2) einkorn wheat, 3) hulled barley, 4) peas, 5) lentils, 6) bitter vetch, 7) chick peas, and 8) flax.

- Farming employs more than 24 million American workers (17% of the total workforce).

- Fast food companies, the movie industry, and theme parks have a long and financially lucrative relationship. The companies seek to promote and "product place" one another for incredible profit. For example, Frito Lay sponsors the California Screamin' roller coaster at Disneyland, and movies intentionally feature a type of fast food (e.g., Pizza Hut in Wayne's World).

- Fat content is not always a good measure of cholesterol content. For example, the liver and other organs are low in fat but very high in cholesterol.

- Fats from junk food trigger the brain to want more food. This effect can last for several days.

- Female cockroaches that ate junk food in a research study became fatter and took longer to reproduce than cockroaches that ate a healthier diet.

- Fennel can be useful for indigestion and spasms of the digestive tract

- Fennel contains the antioxidant flavonoid quercetin

- Food, especially eating meat, has been a central question of Christian history. Many theologians argue that the vegetarian diet is the most compatible with Christian values, such as mercy and compassion.

- Foods rich in fat and sugar can supercharge the brain's reward system, which can overpower the brain's ability to tell an individual to stop eating. The drug rimonabant, which reduces cravings in tobacco users, can also reduce the desire for food, but it has dangerous side effects.

- For 3,000 years, natural liquorice was used as medicine to treat ulcers, sore throats, coughs, and other diseases. The first liquorice "candy" was an attempt to disguise the bitter flavour of the medicine, though now most American liquorice "candy" does not have liquorice's historic therapeutic qualities.

- For a delicious, creamy salad dressing, mix together avocado and fresh carrot juice.

- For a natural breath freshener, try a sprig of parsley

- For best juicing results, use fresh crisp, precooled vegetables. If you need to freeze fresh produce, use frozen produce within 2 to 3 months for best juice flavour.

- For every $1 spent on food, farmers get less than 12 cents for the raw product.

- For maximum nutritional benefits, seeds should be eaten raw.

- For the potassium! (Although it is present in bananas, potassium is the predominant nutrient among most all fruits and vegetables.)

- Form leafy veggies into a compact ball or roll before inserting them into the juicer's feed chute to keep individual leaves from getting stuck between the juicer's feed chute and the plunger that is used to push the food down.

- Fortune cookies were invented in 1916 by George Jung, a Los Angeles noodle maker.

- Forty percent of new cases of anorexia are in girls between the ages of 15 and 19.

- Founded in 1927, 7-Eleven was once called Tote'm stores since customers "toted away" what they bought. In 1946, the name was changed to 7-Eleven to reflect its original hours of operation, 7 a.m. to 11 p.m. 7-Eleven now sells about 144 million Slurpees, 33 million gallons of fountain drinks, 100 million hot dogs, and 60 million donuts and pastries per year.

- Francois Pelletier de la Salle first discovered cholesterol in solid form in gallstones in 1769. It was named "cholesterol" in 1815 by chemist Eugene Chevreul.

- French fried potatoes are the most often eaten vegetable in America.

- French fries are the single most popular fast food in America. In 1970, French fries surpassed regular potato sales in the United States. In 2004, Americans ate 7.5 billion pounds of frozen French fries.

- French philosopher Voltaire used the antiquity of Hinduism to launch a devastating blow to the Bible's claims of dominance and acknowledged that the Hindus' treatment of animals represented a "shaming alternative to the viciousness of European imperialists."

- Fresh beans contain vitamin A, B-complex vitamins, calcium and potassium

- Fried chicken is the most popular meal ordered in sit-down restaurants in the US. The next in popularity are: roast beef, spaghetti, turkey, baked ham, and fried shrimp.

- Fritz Haber (December 1868—January 1934) co-developed with Carl Bosch the process of ammonia synthesis, which is known today as the "Haber Synthesis." While his work led to the production of nitrogen fertilizer, which has helped to feed billions of people (the entire global population, in fact), he also contributed to human destruction with his involvement in chemical agents during WWI.

- Fruit farming began sometime between 6000 and 3000 B.C. Figs were one of the first cultivated fruit crops.

- Full-time homemakers who never worked outside the home are more likely to become obese than women who are married, had kids, and worked outside the home. They were also more likely to report poor health. Researchers believe the lifestyle of the homemaker leads to the risk of obesity and poor health.

"He who takes medicine and neglects to diet wastes the skill of his doctors."

~Chinese Proverb

CHAPTER 7

G- LIFESTYLE

- German chocolate cake was named after Sam German, an American, and did not originate in Germany.

- Gestational diabetes occurs in about 200,000 or 7% of U.S. pregnancies annually.

- Gibbons prefer to eat fruits twice a day. It normally loves to eat ripe, sugary, juicy fruits like figs.

- Girls are developing breasts at younger and younger ages. Researchers point to increasing rates of obesity as a major cause. Specifically, African American girls start getting breasts at 8 years 10 months on average, compared to 9 years 4 months for Hispanic girls and 9 years 8 months among white and Asian girls.

- Girls with ADHD and PTSD are at an increased risk for developing eating disorders and depression. Additionally, studies show that girls in foster care are at an increased risk for developing an eating disorder.

- Global warming may redefine wine growing in the future. Even tiny temperature changes can dramatically change the quality of wine.

- global warming potential increased demand for organic food may compromise the quality of organic farms

- Globally, more than 1.4 billion adults were overweight in 2008. More than half a billion were obese. The World Health Organization estimates 2.3 billion adults will be overweight by 2015 and has declared obesity a worldwide epidemic.

- Globally, over 40 million preschool children were overweight in 2007.

- Good quality juicers can run anywhere from $100–$500. The most expensive juicer is the original Norwalk hydraulic press juicer for $2,495.

- Goulash, a beef soup, originated in Hungary in the 9th century AD.

- Grains of popcorn around 1,000 years old have been found in tombs in Peru. The kernels are so well preserved that they can still be popped.

- Grapefruit can actually react negatively

- Grapefruit can actually react negatively with lots of drugs including cholesterol-lowering medications.

- Grapes are the fruit of a woody grape vine. About 71% of grapes are used for wine. 27% are used as fresh fruit, and 2% are used as dried fruit.

- Grapes are the only fruit that are capable of producing the proper nutrition for the yeast on its skin and sugar in its juice to ferment naturally.

- Grapes do not ripen once plucked

- Grapes explode when you put them in the microwave. You have been warned!

- Greece is the only country in the world that has perpetuated up to the present the ancient tradition of adding a tree resin to wine to give it a unique sappy taste. Most non-Greeks assert this type of Greek wine or retsina wine is an acquired taste and should be served very cold.

- Green beans are diuretic and may be used to treat diabetes

- Green fruits help make your bones and teeth strong.

- Green juice is rich in chlorophyll, which helps the body detoxify and circulate oxygen. It also balances the body's pH by reducing acidity. Low-grade acidosis can zap energy and contribute to many health problems, such as kidney stones.

- Green tea is full of antioxidants which, when added to water, can help boost the health of plants.

- Green tea Unlike black and oolong teas, green tea is minimally processed

- Green-tipped bananas are better for your health than over-ripe bananas.

- Grocers don't have to tell you where your salad comes from.

- Grown in Egypt since at least 2780 B.C., Radishes were originally black

- Guinea pig farms can be found in Peru and other Latin American countries. In Peru, about 65 million guinea pigs are eaten every year.

"Today, more than 95% of all chronic disease is caused by food choice, toxic food ingredients, nutritional deficiencies and lack of physical exercise."

~Mike Adams

CHAPTER 8

H- LIFESTYLE

- Haggis, the national dish of Scotland: take the heart, liver, lungs, and small intestine of a calf or sheep, boil them in the stomach of the animal, season with salt, pepper and onions, add suet and oatmeal. Enjoy!

- Hamburgers are not served in India out of respect for Hindu religious beliefs, and beer is served at McDonald's in Germany.

- Hard-working boy: Dark chocolate increases blood flow to the brain

- Health is related to the word "wholeness"

- Healthy diet It's more important for children to eat a wide range of healthy food than to eat organically. Most paediatricians note that what's more important than buying organic food is that children are eating a wide range of fruits, vegetables, whole grains, and low-fat milk.

- Healthy popcorn In its true form, popcorn is a healthy snack, even a super food

- Heart beat Anorexia causes an abnormally slow heart rate

- Henry A. Wallace (October 7, 1888—November 18, 1965) was Secretary of Agriculture and supported government intervention in farming practices. For example, he ordered slaughtering pigs and ploughing up cotton fields in rural America to help increase the price of these commodities in order to help the economic situation of American farmers.

- Hershey's Kisses were first produced in 1907 and were shaped like a square. A new machine in 1921 gave them their current shape

- Hershey's produces over 80 million chocolate Kisses--every day.

- Hershey's Kisses are called that because the machine that makes them looks like it's kissing the conveyor belt.

- High cholesterol can be genetic. In fact, an inherited genetic condition called familial hypercholesterolemia causes very high LDL cholesterol levels, even at a young age.

- High cholesterol is directly linked to heart disease, which is the #1 killer of men and women in the United States. Each year, over one million Americans have heart attacks and approximately half of a million people die from heart disease.

- High cholesterol itself typically does not have any symptoms, so many people are unaware they are at risk for heart attacks, strokes, and other heart diseases. A simple blood test can determine a person's total cholesterol level. The National Cholesterol Education Program recommends that all adults have their levels checked every five years.

- High-density lipoproteins (HDLs) are typically labelled "good" cholesterol because they have more protein than fat and, instead of ferrying cholesterol around the body as LDL does, HDL sucks up as much excess cholesterol as it can and takes it back to the liver.

- Higher-income women are less likely to be obese than low-income women.

- High-fructose corn syrup (which tricks your body into wanting to eat more and to store more fat) first appeared in 1967, and the average American now consumes 63 pounds of it a year. It is ubiquitous in fast foods.

- Hippocrates, widely considered the father of medicine, includes wine in almost every one of his recorded remedies. He used it for cooling fevers, as a diuretic, as a general antiseptic, and to help convalescence.

- Historically, tea has been viewed as a health drink. Recent studies suggest that tea, especially green tea, helps reduce some forms of cancer, helps bad breath, reduces the risk of cardiovascular disease, reduces blood pressure, helps with weight control, kills bacteria and virus, acts as an anti-inflammatory, and has neuroprotective power.

- Honey is the only food that doesn't spoil.

- Hostess makes 500 million Twinkies a year.

- Hostess Twinkies were invented in 1931 by James Dewar, manager of Continental Bakeries' Chicago factory. He envisioned the product as a way of using the company's thousands of shortcake pans which were otherwise employed only during the strawberry season. Originally called Little Shortcake Fingers, they were renamed Twinkie Fingers, and finally "Twinkies."

- Huckleberries are well liked by lots of mammals such as bears and humans.

"It is easier to change a man's religion than to change his diet."

— Margaret Mead

CHAPTER 9

I- LIFESTYLE

- Iceland consumes more Coca-Cola per capita than any other nation.

- If a child's parents are overweight or obese, a child has an 80% chance of becoming overweight as well.

- If actors are required to drink whisky in a film or TV scene, they often are just drinking watered-down tea instead, which looks the same as whisky.

- If all the morbidly obese people in the U.S. lived in one state, it would have the 12th highest population in the country, with a population greater than that of Virginia.

- If someone held cholesterol in his hand, it would look like a waxy substance that had been scraped from a whitish-yellow candle.

- If there were 100 adults in a room together, 67 of them would be overweight or obese.

- If you put a raisin in a glass of champagne, it will keep floating to the top and sinking to the bottom.

- Improved nutrition (as well as vaccinations and antibiotics) has extended the average U.S. lifespan from 30 to 40 years old in the early twentieth century to 70 to 80 years old today.

- In 1715, Dutch coffee merchants presented the influential King of France, Louis XIV, with a coffee tree of his own. Millions and millions of trees have sprung from that single tree, thanks in part to Chevalier Gabriel Mathieu de Clieu, who stole some cuttings from the tree and began cultivating coffee on Martinique in the Caribbean.

Within 50 years, there were over 20 million trees on Martinique and neighbouring islands.

- In 1830, it took about 250 to 300 labour hours to produce 100 bushels (5 acres) of wheat. In 1975, it took just 3¾ hours.

- In 1860, 'Godey's Lady's Book' advised US women to cook tomatoes for at least 3 hours.

- In 1875, Swiss Daniel Peter discovered a way of mixing condensed milk, manufactured by his friend Henri Nestlé, with chocolate to create the first milk chocolate.

- In 1879, Swiss Rodolphe Lindt discovered couching, an essential process in refining chocolate. He discovered it by accident when his assistant left a machine running all night.

- In 1884, the Aerated Bread Company turned one of their unused rooms into a tearoom. The idea was extremely popular. Tearooms gave a woman a proper place to gather outside the house without a male escort and keep her reputation intact.

- In 1889, Oskar Minkowski (1858-191931) discovered the link between diabetes and the pancreas (pan - "all" + kreas - "flesh") when a dog from which he removed the pancreas developed diabetes.

- In 1890-99 the average consumption of commercial fertilizer was 1,845,900 tons per year. From 1980-89 it was 47,411,166 tons per year.

- In 1891, William Wrigley Jr. began selling soap in Chicago. To increase sales, he gave away gum to his customers. When his gum became a hit, he decided to make and sell the now popular gum, which was later included in rations for soldiers.

- In 1926, when a Los Angeles restaurant owner with the all-American name of Bob Cobb was looking for a way to use up leftovers, he threw together some avocado, celery, tomato, chives, watercress, hard-boiled eggs, chicken, bacon, and Roquefort cheese, and named it after himself: Cobb salad.

- In 1949, Forrest Raffel and his younger brother Leroy created a restaurant that sold roast beef sandwiches. They spelled out the initials "Raffel Brothers (RB) to create the name "Arby's."

- In 1949, Richard and Maurice McDonald opened the first McDonald's restaurant in San Bernardino, California: the McDonald Brothers Burger Bar Drive-In.

- In 1954, the number of tractors on farms surpassed the number of horses and mules for the first time.

- In 1965, a college student named Fred De Luca and family friend Dr. Peter Buck started Subway in Bridgeport, Connecticut. The first restaurant was called Pete's Super Submarines. Subway currently is located in 87 countries.

- In 1970, Americans spent about $6 billion on fast food. In 2006, the spending rose to nearly $142 billion.

- In 1979, in what has become known as the "Twinkie Defense," Daniel White said he killed San Francisco mayor George Moscone and Harvey Milk because he ate too much junk food, such as Twinkies, candy bars, and cupcakes, which caused a chemical imbalance in his brain. He was still convicted and, in 1981, Congress outlawed the "Twinkie Defense."

- In 1988, Italian women started one of the first female organizations devoted to wine, the Le Donne del Vino. Its goal is to encourage and promote women's role in the Italian wine industry.

- In 1990, Congress passed the Organic Foods Production Act (OFPA), which required the U.S. Department of Agriculture (USDA) to develop national standards for organically produced agricultural products.

- In 1995, before television was common in Fiji, Fijians thought the ideal body shape was round, plump, and soft. After three years of watching American shows such as Melrose Place and Beverley Hills 90210, girls in Fiji began developing eating disorders. Fijian females who watched TV three or more hours a night were 50% more likely to feel "too big" or "too fat" than those who watched less TV.

- In 1995, KFC sold 11 pieces of chicken for every man, woman and child in the US.

- In 2000, airlines spent $275 million on 350 million additional gallons of fuel to compensate for the additional weight of their passengers.

- In 2002, Marshall Field's in Chicago made the largest box of chocolate. It had 90,090 Frango mint chocolates and weighed a whopping 3,326 pounds.

- In 2004, PETA released a video taken at Pilgrim's Pride, a chicken supplier to fast food restaurants, which showed intense animal cruelty.

- In 2005, Advertising Age cited Ronald McDonald as the number two top-10 advertising icon of the twentieth century. The Marlboro Man was number one.

- In 2005, the total value of the worldwide tea market was over $20 billion.

- In 2006, the average American farmer grew enough food for 144 other people. In 1940, the average farmer grew food for 19 other people (which was close to enough food).

- In 2007, just 187,816 of the 2.2 million farms in the United States accounted for 63% of sales of agricultural products, marking a trend toward the concentration in agricultural production.

- In 2011, Americans consumed over 65 billion servings of tea, which is approximately 3 billion gallons. An estimated 85% of all tea was black tea, 14% was green tea, and the rest was oolong and white teas.

- In 2012, 17 million farmers in 28 countries planted 170 million hectares of biotech crops.

- In 2012, the Los Angeles city council unanimously approved a resolution that all Mondays in the City of Angels will be meatless. The measure is part of an international campaign to reduce the consumption of meat for health and environmental reason.

- In 2012, U.S. farms and ranches spent $329 billion to produce $388 billion in goods.

- In 2013, Mexico overtook the United States as the most obese nation. Overall, 32.8% of Mexican adults are obese, compared to 31.8% of American adults.

- In a Department of Agriculture study, researchers analysed 12 fruits and found that 90% of the antioxidant activity was in the juice rather than the fibre.

- In a small study at Indiana University, cyclists who drank chocolate milk after a workout had less fatigue and scored higher on endurance tests than those who had a sports drink.

- In A.D. 644, Arab scientists developed a windmill to pump water for irrigation. By the year 1000, Arabs introduced fertilizers to enrich farm soil.

- In an authentic Chinese meal, the last course is soup because it allows the roast duck entree to "swim" toward digestion.

- In ancient Egypt, the ability to store wine until maturity was considered alchemy and was the privilege of only the pharaohs.

- In ancient Greece, a dinner host would take the first sip of wine to assure guests the wine was not poisoned, hence the phrase "drinking to one's health." "Toasting" started in ancient Rome when the Romans continued the Greek tradition but started dropping a piece of toasted bread into each wine glass to temper undesirable tastes or excessive acidity.

- In ancient times, people would make popcorn by heating sand in a fire and then stirring kernels of popcorn in the hot sand.

- In Japan meat from the 'Fugu' or spiny puffer fish is considered a rare delicacy, however the liver and intestines contain a powerful neuro-toxin and the slightest contamination during preparation can be deadly. Restaurants who serve fugu must have 'Fugu certified' chefs. In Japan about one hundred people on average die annually from fugu poisoning.

- In many parts of the world, tea is an important part of the day and an expression of hospitality.

- In Mayan civilization, cacao(cocoa) beans were the currency, and counterfeiting cacao beans out of painted clay had become a thriving industry. Goods could be priced in units of cacao: a slave cost 100 beans, the services of a prostitute cost 10 beans, and a turkey cost 20 beans. While the Spanish conquistadors horded gold, the Mesoamericans horded cacao beans. In some parts of Latin America, the beans were used as a currency as late as the 19th century.

- In medieval Europe, leeches were commonly used to treat babies' illnesses. For example, leeches were placed on a baby's windpipe for croup. Additionally, teething babies were commonly purged or bled.

- In Morocco, it is the man's job to pour the tea. He holds the long spouted pot high above the glass while pouring so that each glass of tea has a slightly frothy head to it.

- In most people, 60%-70% of their cholesterol is carried in LDL particles, which are considered "bad" cholesterol. LDL particles are not all "bad," however, because they act as ferries, taking cholesterol to parts of the body that need it. LDL cholesterol becomes "bad" if there is too much in the body—in which case, it starts depositing cholesterol into the blood stream.

- In movie theatres, for every dollar spent on popcorn, about 90 cents is profit.

- In November 2004, the fast food chain Hardee's introduced the Monster Thickburger. It has 1,420 calories and 107 grams of fat. Fries and soda would add 900 more calories—making it a 2,000 calorie meal, more than the number of calories nutritionists recommend for an entire day for an adult. Food proportion sizes have consistently increased since the late 1970s.

- In Oaxaca, Mexico, healers called curanderos use chocolate to treat several illnesses such as bronchitis. In some regions, children drink chocolate in the morning to ward off scorpion and bee stings.

- In one study, 10 pesticides were found on conventional spinach and 9 were found on celery. Bell peppers had the most, with 39 overall pesticides.

- In one year, the world can produce 3 million tons of cacao, less than half the coffee crop.

- In parts of the world where pesticide is not available, over 1/3 of the food is eaten by pests—whereas in the Western world, where pesticides are used, the loss is reduced by 41%.

- In the 19th century British sailors ate limes to prevent Scurvy

- In the 20th century, English schoolmasters recommended that students become vegetarians as a way to curb their "appetites for self-abuse."

- In the ancient Mayan civilization, humans were often sacrificed to guarantee a good cacao harvest. First, the prisoner was forced to drink a cup of chocolate, which sometimes was spiked with blood because the Maya believed it would convert the victim's heart into a cacao pod.

- In the early 1900s, Mary Isabel Fraser visited China and brought back seeds to New Zealand. She grew the first crop of kiwi in 1910. Today, New Zealand produces 1/3 of the world's supply of kiwi.

- In the film Psycho, Alfred Hitchcock used Bosco chocolate syrup for blood in the famous shower scene.

- In the late 1990s, websites called pro-ana (pro-anorexia) and pro-mia (pro-bulimia) were created for anorexics and bulimics to connect with one another. Many people on these sites deny that anorexia and bulimia are disorders and instead claim they are merely a lifestyle choice.

- In the middle Ages, the greatest and most innovative winemakers of the day were monastic orders. The Cistercians and Benedictines were particularly apt winemakers, and they are said to have actually tasted the earth to discover how the soil changed from place to place. Their findings are still important today.

- In the U.S., 1–2% of the female population and 0.1–0.2 % of males suffer from anorexia.

- In the United States and other developed countries, most livestock is raised on large factory farms called concentrated animal feeding operations, or CAFOs. The largest CAFOs house poultry and contain more than 125,000 chickens at one time.

- In the United States, it is estimated that every adult unconsciously consumes one pound of insects each year due to garden produce, poor restaurant and home hygiene, and commercial foods for which the USDA allows a certain amount of insect fragments. Peanut butter, for example, is allowed to have 30 insect fragments per 100 grams.

- In the United States, lettuce is the second most popular fresh vegetable.

- In the United States, September 29 is celebrated as National Coffee Day. In Costa Rica, it's September 12; in Ireland, it's September 19; and in Japan, it's October 1.

- In the United States, the South and Northeast have the greatest concentration of tea drinkers.

- In the whole of the Biblical Old Testament, only the Book of Jonah has no reference to the vine or wine.

- In Tibet, a common drink is butter tea – it is made from yak butter, salt, and tea.

- In women, diabetes impacts oestrogen levels, menstrual and ovulation cycles, and sexual desire.

- Including fruit and vegetables in one's daily diet can lessen the chances of miscarriage by almost half of the frequency, says a new research in London.

- Including fruit and vegetables in one's daily diet can lessen the chances of miscarriage by almost half of the frequency, says a new research in London.

- India has the world's highest diabetes population with over 35 million people with diabetes. By 2025, this number is expected to swell to 70 million, meaning every fifth diabetic in the world would be Indian.

- Individuals who have inherited other genetic syndromes (Down's syndrome, myotonic syndrome, Turner's syndrome) are also at risk of developing diabetes.

- Individuals with an "apple" body shape are at greater risk for diabetes than are those with "pear" body shapes.

- Individuals with diabetes are more likely to die from a heart attack than those who don't have diabetes.

- Individuals with diabetes are more susceptible to complications of flu and pneumonia and are six times more likely to be hospitalized for these problems than non-diabetics. According to the Centres for Disease Control, 10,000-30,000 people with diabetes die each year from flu and pneumonia.

- Inhaled insulin is an emerging twenty-first century option for people with Type 1 diabetes. Companies are also working on an insulin tablet that can be given under the tongue.

- In-n-Out Burger is one of the few fast food restaurants that actually slice each potato by hand shortly before it is placed in the deep fryer.

- Insects such as termites and ants provide 10% of the protein consumed worldwide. Where insects are an integral part of a diet, they contribute as much as 40% of protein.

- Insulin in the 1920s was initially extracted from the pancreas of a cow (bovine) or pig (porcine). Today's insulin are created in the lab, cultured from bacteria and yeast through recombinant DNA.

- Insulin was coined from the Latin insula ("island") because the hormone is secreted by the Islets of Langerhans in the pancreas.

- Irish cream and Hazelnut are the most popular whole bean coffee flavourings.

- Ironically, the original actor who played Ronald McDonald, Jeff Juliano, is now a vegetarian.

- It is believed ALL citrus fruits derived from the Chinese orange.

- It is estimated that 20–40% of models suffer from some type of eating disorder. Some groups are urging the fashion industry to ban the use of size "0" models. Size 0 usually corresponds to someone who has a Body Mass Index (BMI) below 18.5. An adult who has a BMI between 18.5 and 24.9 is considered to be at a healthy weight. An adult with a BMI of 25.0-29.9 is considered overweight. An adult with a BMI of 30 or higher is considered obese.

- It is traditional to first serve lighter wines and then move to heavier wines throughout a meal. Additionally, white wine should be served before red, younger wine before older and dry wine before sweet.

- It is widely believed that iced tea was invented in 1904 at the St. Louis World Fair by Richard Blechynden, a British tea merchant. However, at least one late 19th century cookbook includes a recipe for iced tea.

- It may also be useful in treating jaundice, cirrhosis, oedema due to high blood pressure, gout, eczema and acne

- It takes 3 to 4 years for a coffee tree to mature. Once it matures, each tree will bear one to two pounds of coffee beans per growing season.

- It takes 3500 calories to make a pound.

- It takes about a half a gallon of water to cook macaroni, and about a gallon to clean the pot.

- It takes approximately 400 cacao beans to make one pound of chocolate.

- It takes around four to 12 years for a tea plant to produce seed. It takes about three years before a new plant is ready to harvest.

"If diet is wrong, medicine is of no use. If diet is correct, medicine is of no need"

-Ancient Ayurvedic proverb

CHAPTER 10

J- LIFESTYLE

- Jain vegetarians will eat dairy but not eggs, honey, or root vegetables.

- Jicama is low in sodium and high in potassium

- Juiced broccoli Juiced broccoli is rich in healthy nutrients. Juiced broccoli can help boost a person's immune system. Broccoli is high in vitamin C, which increases the production of infection-fighting white blood cells. Adding garlic, which contains sulfur-based compounds, also has a powerful immune boosting quality.

- Juiced coconuts provide a rich source of electrolytes. In fact, doctors have used coconut juice to fight dehydration due to dysentery, cholera, and influenza.

- Juiced papaya is an excellent digestive aid. The fruit contains papain, an enzyme that helps digest proteins. Ginger, which helps relax the intestinal tract, and cabbage, which helps clean waste form the stomach and upper bowels, both provide additional digestive power.

- Juicing as way to detox or cleanse the body hasn't been scientifically proven. Researchers note that the body's liver and kidneys detox the body whether a person is juicing or not.

- Juicing avocados and bananas produces a puree rather than a juice, so it is often more effective to blend them instead.

- Junk food became a part of the American diet during the 1920s, but it was through television advertising after WWII that junk food became more ubiquitous and nutritionists subsequently became concerned.

- Junk food is typically defined as foods with little nutritional value that are high in calories, fat, sugar, salt, or caffeine. Junk food can include breakfast cereals, candies, chips, cookies, French fries, gum, hamburgers, hot dogs, ice cream, sodas, and most sweet desserts.

"As I see it, every day you do one of two things: build health or produce disease in yourself."

Adelle Davis

CHAPTER 11

K- LIFESTYLE

- Kale eases lung congestion and is beneficial to the stomach, liver and immune system

- Kale is an excellent source of calcium, iron, vitamins A and C, and chlorophyll

- Ketchup was created for use as a drug, not as a condiment.

- Ketchup was originally a fish sauce originating in the orient

- Kiwi contains twice as much Vitamin C as an orange

- Kiwis were once known as Chinese gooseberries

- Kohlrabi helps to stabilize blood sugar and is therefore useful hypoglycaemia and diabetes

- Kohlrabi, which belongs to the cabbage family, is an excellent source of vitamin C and potassium.

"Most people work hard

and spend their health

trying to achieve wealth.

Then they retire and spend

their wealth trying to get

back their health."

-Kevin Gianni

CHAPTER 12

L- LIFESTYLE

- Large studies in Holland, Denmark, and Austria found the food-poisoning bacterium Campylobacter in 100% of organic chicken flocks, but in only 1/3 of conventional flocks. These studies also found that conventional and organic food had equal rates of contamination with Salmonella and 72% of organic chickens were infected with parasites.

- Late comedian and talk-show host Johnny Carson labelled the hamburger the "McClog the Artery."

- Leaves of raspberry help to regulate menstrual cycles

- Lemon is a good source of Vitamin C-Prevents Scurvy

- Lemons can kill bacteria-as they have high content of acid which makes them suitable for cleaning.

- Lemons contain more sugar than strawberries

- Lemon and lime peels contain D-limonene, an anti-aging compound. The skins of fruits such as kiwi and papaya should be removed prior to juicing, but the skins (peels) of lemons and limes may be left on.

- Leonardo da Vinci argued that humans do not have a God-given right to eat animals

- Lettuce is a member of the sunflower family.

- Light roast coffee Dark coffee has less caffeine than milder roasts. Light roast coffee has more caffeine that dark roast coffee. The longer coffee is roasted, the more caffeine is cooked from the bean.

- Lime oil is useful to cool fevers. It can also stimulate and refresh a tired mind and helps with depression

- Lime oils are often used in perfumes, for cleaning, and for aromatherapy.

- Lipton is the world's best-selling tea brand.

- Livestock farming feeds billions of people and employs 1.3 billion people. That means about 1 in 5 people on Earth work in some aspect of the livestock farming.

- Low cholesterol levels have been associated with higher rates of suicide, violence, Alzheimer's, and accidents. Scientists suggest that cholesterol plays a critical role in neuron signalling and brain structure.

- Lychee seeds are poisonous and should not be eaten.

"In order to change we must be sick and tired of being sick and tired."

~Author Unknown

CHAPTER 13

M- LIFESTYLE

- M&M's were created by Forrest Mars (the son of the founder of Mars, Inc.) and his business partner, Bruce Murrie (the son of the president of the Hershey company). Because both their last names started with "M," they called their new candy M&M's. The original colors were red, yellow, green, orange, brown, and violet.

- Madame du Barry, reputed to be a nymphomaniac, encouraged her lovers to drink chocolate in order to keep up with her.

- Maize (corn) is the second largest crop in the world, and the largest in the United States. Popcorn is approximately two one-thousandths percent of the total crop.

- Major risk factors that increase high LDL levels include cigarette smoking, high blood pressure, low HDL cholesterol (below 40 mg/dL), family history of early heart disease, obesity, and age (men: 45 years or older, women: 55 years or older).

- Mangoes are the most favourite and number 1 fruit in the world.

- Many consumers and winemakers argue that genetically engineered wine would not only lead to uniformity but would also compromise the traditional romance and mystique associated with wine.

- Many nutritionists point to high fructose corn syrup as a major culprit in the nation's obesity crisis. The inexpensive sweetener flooded the American food supply in the early 1980s, about the same time that the nation's obesity rate began to skyrocket.

- Many organic farmers tend to move away from monocultures, where crops are farmed in single-species plots. Crop rotations and mixed planting are much better for the soil and environment.

- Many parents during the Roman empire who were influenced by doctors such as Soranus and Galen often denied their babies colostrum (protein-rich breast milk) believing it was too thick and not good for the child's digestion. They regularly gave their babies to a wet-nurse (though the mother's milk was usually the best) and were likely to wean their babies onto foods that lacked adequate nutrition, such as diluted cereals and mixtures of honey or wine with softened bread.

- Many vegetarians avoid meat because they ethically object to animal cruelty. For example, when stunners aren't effective on hogs, they are sometimes sent to the scalding tanks, meant to soften the skin of dead pigs, while they are still alive and conscious.

- Many years ago explorers used watermelons to carry water on long expeditions

- Marriage therapist Andrew G. Marshall suggests stopping in the middle of love-making to have tea and talk to each other. The idea is that sex, which used to last 15 minutes, can now last an hour and half and allows partners to share intimate moments.

- Mars, Inc, claims that the 3 Musketeers bar was named after its original composition: three pieces and three flavours: vanilla, chocolate, and strawberry. When the price of strawberries rose, the company dropped them as an ingredient in the chocolate bar.

- Mayans used chocolate in baptisms and in marriage ceremonies. It was also sometimes used in the place of blood during ceremonies. Mayan emperors were often buried with jars of chocolate by their side.

- McDonald's is Brazil's largest employer.

- McDonald's is one of the largest owners of real estate in the world and it earns the majority of its profits from collecting rent, not from selling food.

- McDonald's is the largest purchaser of beef, pork, and potatoes and the second largest purchaser of chicken in the world. Its annual orders for french fries constitute 7.5% of America's entire potato crop.

- Men have a higher risk of death from diabetes than women.

- Men with diabetes are at a greater risk for erectile dysfunction (ED) than non-diabetic men. Approximately 50-60% of men with diabetes over the age of 50 have problems with ED. Additionally, ED becomes a problem for diabetic men about 10 to 15 years earlier than a non-diabetic man.

- Microwave popcorn was invented in 1945.An American electronics expert, Perry Spencer, invented microwave popcorn. When he paused in front of a power tube called a magnetron in 1945, he felt a "weird" feeling and noticed that the tube had melted chocolate candy bar he had in his pocket. He decided to see if it would pop popcorn, which it did.

- Middle-aged adults have higher rates of obesity (39.5%) than younger (30.3%) and older (35.4%) adults.

- Minerals constitute 4% of our body weight. Unlike carbohydrates, fats, and proteins, they do not furnish energy. Minerals include calcium, iron, and sodium.

- Mississippi has the highest rate of obesity in the country at 34.9%. Colorado is the thinnest state in the nation with a 20.7% obesity rate.

- Monsanto Company is the leading producing of genetically engineered (GE) seed.

- More than $2 billion of candy is sold for Halloween, more than any other holiday.

- More than 100 agricultural crops in the U.S. are pollinated by bees. In fact, one out of three bites of food people eat is thanks to honeybees.

- More than 200 cups of tea can be brewed from one pound of loose tea leaves.

- More than 200 million boxes of Cracker Jack caramel-coated popcorn are consumed every year in the U.S. alone.

- More than 300 banana-related accidents happened in Britain in 2001 mostly involving people slipping on skins.

- More than 6,000 different kinds of apples are grown around the world. The biggest producer is China, followed by the United States, Iran, Turkey, Russia, Italy, and India.

- Most Americans (90%) do not eat the U.S. daily recommended amount of fresh fruits and veggies. Juicing can help a person meet the daily recommendation in one drink

- Most concerns about genetically modified crops fall into three categories: 1) environmental hazards, 2) human health risks, and 3) economic concerns.

- Most epinephrine needles are not long enough to be effective on obese people. Epinephrine works best when injected into the muscle. When it is injected into the fat layer of the skin, it takes longer to reach the bloodstream.

- Most fashion models are thinner than 98% of American women. The average American woman is 5'4" and weighs 140 pounds. The average model is 5'11" and weighs 117 pounds.

- Most likely due to poor nutrition as children, many Greeks and Romans were shorter than people today. Men from Pompeii, for example, averaged 5 ft. 5-½ in. and women averaged 5 ft. 2 in.

- Most of the world's tea is grown in mountain areas 3,000-7,000 feet above sea level and between the Tropic of Cancer and the Tropic of Capricorn. Tea-producing countries include Argentina, China, India, Indonesia, Kenya Malawi, Sri Lanka, and Tanzania.

- Most physicians do not recommend using juicing as an extreme weight loss measure. Research shows that adding protein is essential to preserving muscle mass during weight loss. Additionally, at the end of an extreme diet, the body's metabolism may have temporarily slowed, which makes the body more prone to building fat cells.

- Most wine is served in a glass that has a gently curved rim at the top to help contain the aromas in the glass. The thinner the glass and the finer the rim, the better. A flaring, trumpet-shaped class dissipates the aromas.

- Most wines are designed to be consumed within a few years of production

- Motecuhzoma Xocoyotzin (Montezuma II), the 9th emperor of the Aztecs, was one of the most wealthy and powerful men in the world. He was also known as The Chocolate King. At the height of his power, he had a stash of nearly a billion cacao beans.

- Mothers who eat junk food while pregnant or breast-feeding have children who are prone to obesity throughout life. The children are also more prone to diabetes, raised cholesterol, and high blood fat.

- Mustard greens are an excellent anticancer vegetable

"True healthcare reform starts in your kitchen, not with governments"

~Anonymous

CHAPTER 14

N- LIFESTYLE

- Native Americans not only ate popcorn, but they made beer and soup out of it too.

- Native Americans would use dried herbs and spices and even chili as popcorn flavourings.

- Nazis would use chocolate to lure Jews onto cattle cars destined for concentration camps.

- Nearly 10 million females and 1 million males have a form of anorexia or bulimia in the United States. Millions more are struggling with compulsive eating disorder. Additionally, over 70 million people worldwide struggle with an eating disorder.

- Nearly 14% of gay men suffer from bulimia and over 20% suffer from anorexia. Scientists believe, however, that such high numbers for homosexuals may be due to their being more comfortable admitting to an eating disorder and seeking treatment, not that homosexuality is a factor in developing an eating disorder.

- Nearly 4 million Americans weigh more than 300 pounds.

- Nearly all cacao trees grow within 20 degrees of the equator, and 75% grow within 8 degrees of either side of it. Cacao trees grow in three main regions: West Africa, South and Central America, and Southeast Asia/Oceania.

- Nebraska produces an estimated 250 million pounds of popcorn per year—more than any other state. This is equivalent to a quarter of all the popcorn the United States produces every year.

- Ninety percent of modern cacao is made from a type of cacao called forastero (foreigner). However, before the 1800s, cacao was made from a type of bean called criollo. Even though forastero does not taste as good as criollo, it is easier to grow.

- No one really knows when donuts were invented or who invented them.

- Noble rot, or portraiture noble, is a benign type of grape fungus that can actually sweeten some types of wine.

- Non-organic peanut butters are high in pesticides and fungus and contain aflatoxin, a potent carcinogenic mold.

- North Korea is one of the few countries where Coca-Cola and Pepsi-Cola are not readily available

- Not all wines improve with time. In fact, a vast majority of wines produced are ready to drink and do not have much potential for aging. Only a rare few will last longer than a decade.

- Nutmeg is extremely poisonous if injected intravenously

- Nutrients are divided into two major groups: macronutrients and micronutrients. Macronutrients include protein, carbohydrates, water, and fats. Micronutrients are vitamins and minerals.

- Nutrition" is derived from "nourish," which is from the Latin nutrire, meaning to feed, nurse, support, and preserve--literally, "she who gives suck." Essentially, nutrition refers to the variety of ways the body makes use of food.

"Let food be thy medicine

and medicine be thy food"

~Hippocrates

CHAPTER 15

O- LIFESTYLE

- Obese children and teens who lose weight are in danger of developing eating disorders, including anorexia and bulimia. These problems may go undiagnosed or disregarded because parents and doctors think, "It's a good thing these teens have lost so much weight."

- Obese children quadruple their risk and overweight children double their risk of developing high blood pressure in adulthood.

- Obese men aged 30–49 are less likely to use a condom.

- Obese men and women reported being significantly less sexually satisfied than the general population

- Obese men are 2½ times more likely to struggle with erectile dysfunction.

- Obese people tend to be less sexually active, but when they are sexually engaged, they are more likely to practice unsafe behaviours.

- Obese people, especially women, are less successful than their slimmer peers. Additionally, larger girls are less likely to go to college, regardless of how well they did in high school. Weight was not nearly as big a factor in the career trajectories of men.

- Obese teens and young adults may be more receptive to TV fast food ads than those who aren't obese. Experts aren't sure what comes first, being receptive to TV fast food ads or obesity.

- Obese women are 70% less likely to use birth control pills and eight times more likely to use less-effective methods, such as withdrawal. Obese women were also less likely to obtain advice about contraceptives.

- Obese women are five times more likely to have met a sexual partner on the Internet and to have an obese partner.

- Obesity and overweight issues are linked to more deaths around the world than underweight issues.

- Obesity can be a side effect of certain disorders, such as Cushing's syndrome, hypothyroidism, neurological disturbances (damage to the hypothalamus), or drugs (steroids, antipsychotic medications, or antidepressants).

- Obesity can cause a condition called "buried penis," in which a penis of normal length is buried below the surface of the pubic skin or within its own excessive shaft skin. This condition can cause other problems, including chronic infections, skin breakdown, and chronic inflammation.

- Obesity can strain muscles in the pelvic area, which can weaken muscles, contributing to vaginal prolapse.

- Obesity has been linked to semi-frequent and episodic migraines

- Obesity is an inflammatory disease. In other words, excess calories cause an immune response, which constantly activates a person's immune system at a low level, contributing to widespread inflammation in the body.

- Obesity is becoming the number one cause of liver cirrhosis and liver failure in kids.

- Obesity is known to be a major risk factor for breast cancer in postmenopausal women. It also may determine the rate of breast cancer cell growth and tumour size.

- Obesity is linked to at least 15 medical conditions, including osteoarthritis, cancer, cardiovascular disease, hypertension, joint-related pain, strokes, and impaired immune response.

- Obesity is linked to not only pancreatic cancer but also to lower survival rates of that cancer.

- Obesity is strongly related to osteoarthritis and knee osteoarthritis. More than 50 million Americans have arthritis, and almost half of them can't perform normal daily activities because of the disease. Rising rates of obesity among people younger than 65 may be the main reason for the rapidly increasing number of knee replacements in the U.S.

- Obesity is the abnormal accumulation of body fat, usually 20% or more over an individual's ideal body weight. Obesity is associated with increased risk of illness, disability, and death.

- Obesity is typically caused by several factors, including excess food consumption, lack of exercise, and genetics.

- Oenophobia is an intense fear or hatred of wine.

- Of all Americans with unhealthy levels of cholesterol, 1 in 7 have what is considered "high" cholesterol, or levels that put them at nearly twice the risk of developing heart disease. "High" cholesterol is defined as 240 mg. per decilitre (mg/dL) and above.

- Of those suffering from an eating disorder, only 1 in 10 will receive treatment. Men are less likely to seek treatment for eating disorders because such disorders are typically perceived as a "woman's disease."

- Okinawans are thought to live longer than any other ethnic group and they have healthier hearts and bones. This is largely due to their cultural practice called Hara Hachi Bu, which means they eat just until they are 80% full. Their diet is rich in complex carbohydrates and plant-based foods and is low in fat. They are also physically active.

- Older mothers lend more chance of obesity to their children than young mothers.

- Olympic swimmer Gary Hall Jr. has Type 1 diabetes. When he was diagnosed, his physician told him to give up swimming. He changed doctors, continued training, and subsequently won a gold medal.

- On a side note: Because bananas are so popular, rainforests are often destroyed to make way for banana plantations.

- On average, patients who have undergone gastric bypass surgery keep off at least 50–60% of excess weight over 5–15 years.

- Once reserved for the elite, chocolate became available to everyone due to the technological advances of the Industrial Revolution. However, as chocolate became increasingly popular in Europe and America, thousands of people were used as slaves to produce cacao.

- One chocolate chip can give a person enough energy to walk 150 feet.

- One hundred years ago, the average person ate less than 10 pounds of sugar per year. Today, the average person in the U.S. eats over 100 pounds per year. Currently, sugar intake represents 50% of a person's carbohydrate intake for the day. According to the World Health Organization (WHO), only 10% of a person's diet should come from sugar.

- One in three farm acres is planted for export.

- One in three U.S. children and teens are overweight or obese.

- One of Louis XV's many mistresses, Madame de Pompadour, became a famous chocolate addict and used it as a treatment for her sexual dysfunctions. The Marquis de Sade, possibly the world's first sexologist, was also hooked on chocolate.

- One of Queen Victoria's ladies in waiting, the Duchess of Bedford, is usually credited with the idea of "English Afternoon Tea." The British invented two kinds of afternoon tea: "Low tea," or afternoon tea served on a low "tea table," and "high tea," which is served on a "high" dining room table.

- One of the first famous vegetarians was the Greek philosopher Pythagoras who lived at the end of the 6th century B.C. In fact, the term "Pythagorean diet" was commonly used for a plant-based diet until the term "vegetarian" was coined in the 19th century.

- One of the most quoted legends about the discovery of wine is the story of Jamsheed a semi-mythical Persian king (who may have been Noah). A woman of his harem tried to take her life with fermented grapes, which were thought to be poisonous. Wine was discovered when she found herself rejuvenated and lively.

- One third of the tap water used for drinking in North America is used to brew daily cups of coffee.

- One ton of grapes make about 60 cases of wine, or 720 bottles. One bottle of wine contains about 2.8 pounds of grapes.

- One way to combat obesity is to eat slowly. It takes the brain 20 minutes to sense that a person is full.

- Onions aid in cellular repair.

- Onions are a rich source of quercetin, a potent antioxidant.

- Onions are an excellent antioxidant, and they contain anti-allergy, antiviral and antihistamine properties.

- Orange fruits help keep your eyes healthy.

- Orange Juice naturally contains a small amount of alcohol.

- Oranges contain antioxidants that help fight the free radicals that damage and age our skin

- Oranges help fight anti-aging

- Orang-utans love mangoes

- Organic farmers can treat fungal diseases with copper solutions. The organic insecticide rotenone is highly neurotoxic to humans, does not readily biodegrade, and rotenone exposure has been linked Parkinson's disease.

- Organic food is food that has been grown or processed without synthetic pesticides, chemical fertilizers, irradiation, industrial solvents, or chemical food additives.

- Organic food is typically more expensive than conventional food, sometimes 50% higher than the same conventionally grown food.

- Organic food labelling standards are based on the percentage of organic ingredients in a product. Products labeled "100% organic" must contain only organically produced ingredients. Products labeled "organic" must contain at least 95% organically produced ingredients. Processed products made with at least 70% organic ingredients may use the phrase "made with organic ingredients."

- Organic foods tend to have higher levels of pathogens than conventionally grown ones because manure is used to fertilize them. For example, E. coli was found in 10% of produce from organic farms, but in only 2% from conventional farms.
- Organic milk is the fastest growing sector in the beverage market.
- Organically reared cows burp up twice as much methane as conventionally reared cattle. Methane is 20 times more powerful a greenhouse gas than CO_2.
- Orthopraxis are obsessed with food quality rather than quantity. They are not so much obsessed with a thin body but personal purity.
- Orville Redenbacher is the #1 best-selling popcorn in the world. Its inventor, Orville, began to grow popping corn in 1919, when he was just 12 years old.
- Osage orange fruits are used to repel cockroaches
- Over 1.42 million pounds of tea are consumed in the U.S. every day.
- Over 250 million people worldwide have type-2 diabetes, constituting more than 90 percent of global diabetes cases. Most people will eventually become disabled or die from the disease.
- Over 3 million tons of tea is produced every year worldwide.
- Over 300,000 deaths in the U.S. a year are attributed to obesity. Obesity is second only to smoking as a cause of premature death in the United States.
- Over 50% of adults in America prefer chocolate to other flavours.
- Over 519 million pounds of tea are imported into the United States each year.
- Over 65% of tea brewed in the United States was prepared using tea bags.

- Overall, men and women have similar rates of obesity. However, 56.6% of black women were obese compared with 37.1% of black men.

- Overweight individuals are more prone to develop diabetes because more fat requires more insulin, fat cells release free fatty acids which interfere with glucose metabolism, and overweight people have fewer available insulin receptors.

- Owing to the nature of cacao butter, chocolate is the only edible substance that melts at around 93° F, just below body temperature. This means that after placing a piece of chocolate on your tongue, it will begin to melt.

- Owning and controlling a farm has historically been linked to status and power, especially in Medieval European agrarian societies. Farm ownership has also been historically linked to types of government (feudalism, democracy, etc.).

"If you can't pronounce it,

don't eat it" ~

Common sense

CHAPTER 16

P- LIFESTYLE

- Parsley contains vitamin A and is a good source of copper and manganese

- Parsley is an ant carcinogen

- Parsley is useful as a digestive aid

- Peanut is the main component of nitro-glycerine

- Peanuts are high in fungus and, often, pesticides.

- Peanuts are one of the ingredients in dynamite.

- Peanuts can be used for a component to make Dynamite.

- Peanuts contain about the same amount of protein as soy and are low in starchy carbohydrates.

- Peanuts contain beneficial protein, but many people are allergic to them and find them hard to digest.

- Pearls melt in vinegar.

- Pear-wood is hard

- People become vegetarians for several reason, including ethical, health, political, environmental, cultural, aesthetic, and economic concerns.

- People living near factory farms often suffer from headaches, nausea, and respiratory distress due to the effects of factory pollution. Factory farms are those that pack hundreds, thousands, and sometimes millions of cows, pigs, chickens into the farms.

- People who feel depressed eat about 55% more chocolate than their non-depressed peers.

- People with extreme anorexia will develop downy body hair that grows on the back, arms, legs, face and neck. This is called lanugo and is the body's attempt to maintain a normal temperature after losing so much fat. This type of hair requires fewer calories to produce than normal hair.

- People with less than a high school degree have the highest obesity rates (32.9%). High school graduates (29.5%) have about the same obesity rates as college dropouts (29.1%). College graduates have the lowest obesity rate at 20.8%.

- Pesticides may be used on organic food as long as they are not synthetic.

- Physicians recommend talking with a health care provider before incorporating juice into a diet to avoid potential food and drug interactions. For example, large amounts of foods high in vitamin K (e.g., spinach and kale) may interact with some anti-blood-clotting medicine.

- Pigs, a common farm animal, are thought to be the 4th most intelligent animal, after chimps, dolphins, and elephants. A group of pigs is called a sounder. Pigs can also run 11 miles per hour, which is faster than a 6-minute mile.

- Pilgrims ate popcorn at the first Thanksgiving dinner.

- Pineapples are berries, just like strawberries and blueberries.

- Pineapples contain an enzyme that is used in blood tests. Fibres in pineapple leaves are used to make rope and a cloth called pino.

- Pineapples used in blood tests

- Plants yield 10 times more protein per acre than meat.

- Plato argued that the minimum drinking age should be 18, and then wine in moderation may be tasted until 31. When a man reaches 40, he may drink as much as he wants to cure the "crabbedness of old age."

- Pollution can be a cause of obesity. Pollution affects our hormones, which control our weight.

- Popcorn has been sold in theatres since 1912. It has been a big money maker not only because popcorn is overpriced, but also because people usually get thirsty and, consequently, buy sodas or water as well.

- Popcorn has more protein than any other cereal grain. It also has more iron than eggs or roast beef. It has more fibre than pretzels or potato chips.

- Popcorn is the official snack of Illinois. Since 1958, there has been an annual "Popcorn Day."

- Popcorn kernels can pop up to 3 feet in the air.

- Popcorn kernels, like those of all cereal, have three major components: the germ or embryo, the endosperm, and the outer hull called the pericarp.

- Popcorn is a healthy snack for diabetics

- Popped corn contains large amounts of protein, vitamins, and minerals. Among other health benefits, popped corn helps build bones and muscle tissues and assists in digestion. It is also rich in antioxidants (polyphenols). Most of the nutrients are found in the "hull" or shell rather than the fluffy, white part. However, popcorn that has too much butter, oil, or salt compromises its health benefits.

- Popped popcorn comes in two shapes: "snowflake" or "mushroom." Because "snowflake" shaped popcorn is bigger, movie theatres typically sell that shape.

- Popular movies about farming include Country (1984), The River (1984), Out of Africa (1985), Giant (1956), and The Big Country (1958).

- Portuguese poet Fernando Pessoa once wrote, "There is no metaphysics on earth like chocolate."

- Pretty Woman Eating chocolate regularly can improve a woman's sex life .According to Italian researchers, women who eat chocolate regularly have a better sex life than those who do not. They also had higher levels of desire, arousal, and satisfaction from sex.

- Proportionally, hash browns have more fat and calories than a cheeseburger or Big Mac.

- Psychiatrist Gerald Russell, who is credited with publishing the first description of bulimia nervosa in 1979, noticed scarring on top of the bulimics' hands due to the teeth rubbing on the hands as the person forces them back into the throat repeatedly. These scars are called "Russell's signs."

- Pumpkin seeds are high in zinc, which is good for the prostate and building the immune system.

- Pumpkins and avocados are fruits not a vegetable.

- Purging causes serious health problems, including severe tooth decay, swollen cheeks and salivary glands, dangerous loss of potassium that can lead to fatal heart problems, and a ruptured oesophagus or stomach. Like anorexia, bulimia also damages the body's organs, including the stomach and kidneys.

- Purple Mangos teen has to be grown in temperatures of above 40 °F (4 °C). If it is grown in temperatures below that, the plants will die.

- Quakers, such as George Cadbury, amassed a great fortune producing drinking chocolate as an alternative to alcohol.

"Time and health are two precious assets that we don't recognize and appreciate until they have been depleted."

~Denis Waitley

CHAPTER 17

R- LIFESTYLE

- Radishes contain vitamin C, potassium and other trace minerals

- Radishes have antibacterial and anti-fungal properties

- Raising beef cattle is the single largest segment of American agriculture. The United States produces more beef than any other country. About 34 million cows are slaughtered in the U.S. each year.

- Raisins are dried grapes. They contain a lot of sugar.

- Raw food dieticians recommend drinking juiced raw vegetables immediately after they are prepared and on an empty stomach. They suggest waiting 10–15 minutes to eat after drinking 8–30 ounces. If you drink more than 30 ounces, they suggest waiting at least 45 minutes before eating. Drinking juice on an empty stomach helps the nutrients to be absorbed more quickly and efficiently.

- Raw juice: Juicing for 2 people and cleaning up takes about 10-15 minutes. Depending on cooking temperature and time, vitamins, antioxidants, and phytonutrients are lost in varying degrees while cooking. Other negative affects of cooking food include the following: 1) proteins become denatured, which renders them useless to the body, 2) water in food evaporates, which leads to the loss of valuable minerals and water-soluble vitamins like vitamins C and B-complex, 3) food reduces in volume but maintains its calorie count, so you end up eating more calories by volume of food than your body needs, 4) food softens, making it easier to eat quickly and overeat, and 5) high heat creates toxins, especially when cooking starches and fats.

- Raw food nutritionists recommend chewing raw juice. When drinking juice, chewing activates the digestive elements in the mouth, which helps assimilate the juice in the body.

- Raw foodists argue that humans are the only mammals that continue to drink milk (and another mammal's milk—the cow's—also something no other mammal does) after being weaned because of the belief that milk is important for calcium. However, plants provide all the calcium the body needs without the health risks of milk. Some of the best sources of calcium are collard greens, kale, spinach, okra, broccoli, and almonds.

- Raw foodists suggest that the leftover pulp from juicing can be put back into the juice or used in cooking, such as muffins or broth.

- Raw pumpkin seeds contain essential fatty acids and beneficial proteins.

- Red Burgundy is made from the Pinot Noir grape and is so difficult to make that winemakers all over the world see it as some kind of Holy Grail.

- Red fruits help keep your heart strong.

- Red wine represents 55% of restaurant wine sales.

- Red wine, typically more than white wine, has antioxidant properties and contains resveratrol, which seems to be important in the cardio-protective effects of wine.

- Red wines are red because fermentation extracts colour from the grape skins. White wines are not fermented with the skins present.

- Reduced blood flow caused by high cholesterol has been linked to sexual disorders. High cholesterol causes fatty deposits that clog blood vessels in the pelvic area, causing erectile dysfunction in men and possibly impacting lubrication in women.

- Reports predict that the global chocolate market will grow to $98.3 billion in 2016 from $83.2 billion in 2010.

- Research has shown that drinking coffee may decrease cognitive decline and neurodegenerative disorders.

- Research notes that people may buy organic food based on psychological effects, such as the "halo effect." In other words, the label "organic" can change perceptions of taste, calories, and value regardless of whether the food is organic or not.

- Research reveals that if a man avoids red meats, it improves the sex appeal of his body odour.

- Research says eating grapefruit in the morning will helps to lose an average of 3.6 pounds. It also protect from diabetes.

- Research shows that genes do affect a person's risk of becoming overweight. One gene in particular, the FTO gene, has the greatest effect.

- Research shows that organic milk and conventionally processed milk have similar levels of contaminants, including growth hormones. The AAP emphasizes that what is important is that children should drink pasteurized milk to reduce the risk of bacterial infection.

- Research shows that smoking lowers good cholesterol (HDL) and raises bad cholesterol (LDL). Researchers found that those who stopped smoking experienced an average increase of approximately 5%, or 2.4 mg/dL, in HDL cholesterol.

- Research shows that stress increases "bad" cholesterol levels. In contrast, the better a person copes with the stress, the higher his "good" cholesterol levels are.

- Research suggests that a "gut germ" transplant may help obese people shed pounds. In other words, obese people may benefit from a thinner person's gut germs because thinner people's intestinal bacteria digest food differently than obese people's do. The gut, where the body processes food, is crucial to weight gain and weight loss.

- Research suggests that dark chocolate boosts memory, attention span, reaction time, and problem-solving skills by increasing blood flow to the brain. Studies have also found that dark chocolate can improve the ability to see in low-contrast situations (such as poor weather) and promote lower blood pressure, which has positive effects on cholesterol levels, platelet function, and insulin sensitivity.

- Research suggests that the increased use of herbicide designed to work with GMOs (and vice versa) is starting to create "super weeds" that resist chemicals.

- Researchers found that every two hours spent watching television was associated with a 14% increase in diabetes risk.

- Researchers have found no link between acne and chocolate. In fact, German researchers suggest that flavonoids in chocolate absorb UV light, which help protect and increase blood flow to the skin, ultimately improving its appearance.

- Researchers note that there is not a significant difference between organic and conventional food in nutritional value, potential allergic reactions, or incidents of Campylobacter infections (a common cause of bacterial foodborne illness). Additionally, studies show that organic food does not significantly taste better than conventional food.

- Researchers suggest that average glucose levels can be higher for diabetic girls with menstrual difficulties. Additionally, girls with menstrual problems also had a higher rate of hospital admissions for diabetic ketoacidosis (DKA).

- Researchers suggest that breast cancer rates in China are rising because of an increase in Western-style junk food and increasing unhealthy lifestyles.

- Researchers worry that increased consumer demand for organic food may lead to larger farms, lowered standards for organic produce, and poorer working conditions for organic farmers.

- Richer, heavier foods usually go well with richer, heavier wines; lighter foods demand light wines. Additionally, red wine typically is served with red meat, white wine with white meat and fish, and sweet wine with desserts.

- Roasted seeds contain damaged fat that can lead to plaque in the arteries

- Romans discovered that mixing lead with wine not only helped preserve wine, but also gave it a sweet taste and succulent texture. Chronic lead poisoning has often been cited as one of the causes of the decline of Rome.

- Rosehip tea Herbal tea has been infused with herbs, spices, or other plant material

- Roughly half of all U.S. advertising directed at children and teens is for food.

- Russian author Leo Tolstoy gave up meat because he was concerned about animal cruelty. He claims that eating meat is unnecessary, leads to animalistic feelings, excites human desires, and encourages "fornication and drunkenness."

- Russians started drinking tea in the 17th century, but because of its high price, it did not become widely popular until the beginning of the 19th century. Tea in Russia has historically been prepared in a samovar, a heated metal container. The samovar keeps tea hot for hours.

"From the bitterness of

disease man learns the

sweetness of health."

~Catalan Proverb

CHAPTER 18

S- LIFESTYLE

- Salt is the most common seasoning mentioned in the Bible. Salt was a vital mineral that was not only essential to life, but also preserved other foods critical for survival. Salt was so important that it was also often used as a form of currency or as a unit of exchange.

- Sapodilla is a uniquely tasted fruit. It had a soft brown flesh which flavours like a sweet mix of brown sugar and root beer.

- Scientists have identified a group of chemicals called saponins in red wine that helps lower cholesterol.

- Scientists predict that there may be 30 million new cases of diabetes in China alone by 2025.

- Scientists suggest that some girls develop anorexia because they are afraid to separate from their parents, particularly their mothers. They develop an eating disorder to halt their sexual development as a way to avoid leaving childhood.

- Second only to Santa Claus, Ronald McDonald is recognized by over 96% of American children

- Seeds had to be scattered by hand until Jethro Tull's seed drill (developed in 1701) made it possible to plant seeds in rows, which could then be easily hoed.

- Self- induced vomiting Purging has severe health risks

- Serving temperatures should be lower for white (45-50 degrees Fahrenheit) than for red wines (50-60 degrees Fahrenheit).

- Seven coffee seeds Baba Budan smuggled the first coffee seeds out of the Middle East

- Several groups have called on organic food producers not to use nanotechnology, which is the process of manipulating matter at the atomic and molecular matter. Some nanotechnology already exists in organic products. For example, Nano Green Sciences sells a nano-pesticide they claim is "organic." Additionally, some personal care products that are promoted as being "organic" also already contain nanoparticles.

- Several researchers argue that a vegetarian diet can feed more people than a meat-based diet. For example, approximately 20,000 pounds of potatoes can be grown on one acre of land. Comparatively, only around 165 pounds of beef can be produced on 1 acre of land.

- Several studies indicate that it would have been biologically impossible for humans to evolve large brains on a raw vegan diet. They conclude that meat-eating was crucial in human evolution.

- Several studies show that a plant-based diet increases the body's metabolism, causing the body to burn calories up to 16% faster than the body would on a meat-based diet for at least the first 3 hours after meals.

- Severe obesity is defined as a body-mass index (BMI) of 35 or greater, or 220 pounds or more.

- Since wine tasting is essentially wine smelling, women tend to be better wine testers because women, particularly of reproductive ages, have a better sense of smell than men.

- Sir John Krebs, former chairman of Britain's Food Standards Agency, claimed in 2002 that "a single cup of coffee contains natural carcinogens equal to at least a year's worth of synthetic carcinogenic residues in the diet."
- Smelling bananas and/or green apples (smelling, not eating) can help you lose weight!
- Smoking can increase diabetes risk by constricting blood vessels, raising blood pressure, and stimulating the release of catecholamines (fight-or-flight hormones), which promote insulin resistance.
- Smoking marijuana cigarettes increases a person's appetite by a whopping 40%.
- Snickers are the most popular candy bar in America, due in part to advertising that highlighted its healthful aspects. In the UK, Snickers was initially named Marathon Bar because "snickers" rhymes with "knickers," a British colloquialism for someone's underwear.
- Solid blocks of tea were used as money in Siberia until the 19th century.
- Some children and pregnant women crave non-nutritive substances, such as paint, plaster, rocks, and dirt. These cravings may suggest the person lacks certain minerals, such as iron.
- Some horticulturists suspect that the banana was the earth's first fruit.
- Some of the healthier fast food choices include Arby's Light Roast Chicken Sandwich (276 calories, 7 grams of fat, 777 mg sodium, 33 mg cholesterol), Burger King's Chunky Chicken Salad (142 calories, 4 grams of fat, 443 mg sodium, 49 mg cholesterol), Wendy's Chili (210 calories, 7 grams of fat, 800 mg sodium, 30 mg cholesterol), and McDonald's Vanilla Shake (310 calories, 5 grams of fat, 170 mg sodium, 25 mg cholesterol).

- Some scholars link the growing popularity of chocolate houses in Europe, such as the Cocoa-Tree Chocolate House on St. James Street in London, with the beginnings of the Enlightenment. That was the drink on the table when 18th-century thinkers started to question long-held verities: the supremacy of the Church, the rights of kings, and potential for improvement in the common man and woman.

- Some vegetarians may not know that rennet is often used to make cheese and, therefore, unknowingly eat it. Rennet is extracted from the inner mucosa of the fourth stomach chamber of slaughtered young, un-weaned calves.

- Someone who was obese as a child can have a harder time losing weight later in life since they may have up to five times as many fat cells as someone who became overweight as an adult.

- South Carolina is the only state that has a major tea plantation. It produces the brand American Classic, which has been the official White House tea since 1987

- Starbuck coffee shops use over 93 million gallons of milk per year. This would be enough to fill 155 Olympic-sized swimming pools. Additionally, they use 2.3 billion paper cups annually.

- Starbucks opened in Seattle in 1971. In 2010, it boasted revenues of $10.7 billion and 16,850 stores in 40 countries, making it the world's top coffee retailer. Starbucks offers over 87,000 possible drink combinations.

- Strawberries and cashews are the only fruits that have their seeds on the outside unlike all other fruits which have their seeds inside

- Strawberries and cashews have seeds outside them

- Strawberries are the only fruit

- Strawberries are the only fruit which grows seeds on the outside.

- Strawberry is not a berry

- Studies have shown that incidence of cancer among conventional farmers, who are routinely exposed to relatively high levels of pesticides, are lower than in the wider population. In the past 50 years, since synthetic chemicals have come into wide use, average life expectancy has increased by more than 7 years.

- Studies have shown that pesticide levels in children's urine were significantly lower if they ate organic diets.

- Studies show that a vegetarian diet could feed more people than a meat-based diet. For example, only around 20% of the corn grown in the United States is eaten by people, with about 80% of the corn eaten by livestock. Additionally, approximately 95% of the oats grown in the U.S are eaten by livestock. Studies show that the number of people who could be fed by the grain and soybeans that are currently fed to U.S. livestock is approximate 1,300,000,000.

- Studies show that breast-fed babies have lower levels of cholesterol as adults. Additionally, breast milk is rich in healthy cholesterol and fats, which help prevent adult heart and central nervous system diseases.

- Studies show that drinking coffee reduces the risk of Alzheimer's disease, Parkinson's disease, heart disease, diabetes mellitus type 2, cirrhosis of the liver, and gout.

- Studies show that men who drink six or more cups of coffee daily decrease their risk of developing prostate cancer by 20%.

- Subsistence farmers are farmers who produce the food they need to survive on a daily basis. They are farmers who raise enough food for themselves and their families. The food is not intended to be sold in a market.

- Sulphur compounds in onions help to detoxify the body.

- Sunlight is a major source of Vitamin D

- Sweet potatoes are also high in sugar and therefore should be used sparingly

- Sweet potatoes are an excellent source of carotenoid antioxidants

- Sweet potatoes are not related to the potato nor the yam--they are actually a member of the morning glory family

- Swirling oxygenates wine and helps release its aromas

"The best and most efficient pharmacy is within your own system."

~Robert C. Peale

CHAPTER 19

T- LIFESTYLE

- TEA: A Chinese emperor discovered tea in 2737 B.C. According to legend, tea was discovered in 2737 B.C. by Chinese Emperor Shen-Ning, known as the "Divine Healer." Purportedly, he discovered the beverage when tea leaves accidentally blew into his pot of boiling water.

- Tea is the most widely consumed beverage in the world, after water.

- Tea is the national drink in Iran and Afghanistan. Green tea is consumed as a thirst quencher, and black tea as a warming beverage. Both of them are prepared with lots of sugars.

- Tea plants need at least 50 inches of rain a year.

- Tea plants thrive in hot, humid climates with high rainfall

- Tea sets in the 18th century typically had numbered spoons to help the host remember which guest needed a refill.

- Tea was a major factor in establishing connections between the East and West. It was also a catalyst for developing new technology, such as faster transport ships.

- Tea was initially sold in coffee houses in England. Only men were allowed to enter coffee houses, which were full of smoke and noise. Finally, in 1717, the Twining family opened the Golden Lyon, a teashop that allowed women. The shop is still open today, and the Twinings company is a prominent English marketer of tea.

- Tea was more popular than coffee in America until King George the III's Stamp Act of 1767 increased taxes. The result was the Boston Tea Party, a rebellion in which

Bostonians dumped the British East India tea cargos into a harbour. From that point, coffee became America's national drink and was emotionally linked with its revolution.

- Television greatly expanded the ability of advertisers to reach children and try to develop brand loyalty early in life. Today the average American child sees more than 10,000 food advertisements each year on television.

- Temperature can affect appetite. A cold person is more likely to eat more food.

- Testosterone may play a significant role in the origins of eating disorders in males. Studies show that males with anorexia may have problems producing testosterone.

- The 4-digit price look-up (PLUs) codes on produce indicate the type of produce. For example, #4011 is code for a standard banana. The number "9" prefix on a PLU indicates an item is organic. For example, #94011 is an organic banana. The number "8" indicates the produce is genetically engineered. For example, #84011 is a genetically engineered banana.

- The 57 on the Heinz ketchup bottle represents the number of varieties of pickles the company once had.

- The Adam's apple is so-called coz of the idea that it was created when the forbidden fruit got stuck in Adam's throat when he swallowed it.

- The agent that gives Twinkies their smooth feel, cellulose gum, is also used in rocket fuel to give it a slightly gelatinous feel.

- The American Dietetic Association (ADA) concludes that a vegetarian or vegan diet is healthier than one that includes meat. They note that vegetarians have lower body mass indices, lower rates of death from ischemic heart disease, lower blood cholesterol levels, lower blood pressure, lower rates of hypertension, type 2 diabetes, and less prostate and colon cancer.

- The American Heart Association recommends a maximum intake of 300 mg. of cholesterol per day for those who have normal levels. Those who already have high cholesterol should eat no more than 200 mg. per day. While eggs are lower in cholesterol than previously thought, one large chicken egg still contains about 185 mg of cholesterol, all of which is contained in the yolk.

- The American Heart Association recommends a maximum of no more than 2 grams of trans fat per day. A person should eat no more than 1,000-3,000 mg of sodium per day. Men need about 2,700 calories a day, while women need about 2,000 per day.

- The amount of caffeine in coffee depends on the type of beans, how they were roasted, and how the coffee was brewed. Typically, a small 8-ounce cup of coffee has between 65 milligrams of caffeine if it's instant and 115 milligrams if it's drip brewed.

- The Arabs discovered coffee, but were jealous of their discovery and refused to allow fertile coffee seeds to leave their country. However a 17th-century Muslim pilgrim, Baba Budan, smuggled seven seeds out of Arabia and planted them in India. It is said that all the world's coffee came from these seven seeds.

- The average American eats an amount of fat equivalent to one whole stick of butter each day.

- The average American/Canadian drinks about 600 sodas a year!

- The average American/Canadian will eat about 11.9 pounds of cereal per year!

- The average ear of corn has eight-hundred kernels arranged in sixteen rows.

- The Aztecs used popcorn during ceremonies. Several young women would dance a "popcorn dance" with popcorn garlands on their heads. They also used popcorn as decoration for ceremonial headdresses, necklaces, and ornaments on statues of their gods.

- The banana plant can grow as high as 20 feet tall. That's as big as a two-story house!

- The Bergerac wine region in southwest France has produced wine since Roman times

- The best way to lose weight is to eat fewer calories and increase exercise. Experts suggest aiming for a weight loss goal of one pound per week.

- The cabbage encloses nearly as much water as watermelon. Watermelon contains 92% water where cabbage is 90% and carrots are 87%

- The cacao bean naturally contains almost 300 different flavours and 400 separate aromas.

- The Catholic Church once associated chocolate with heretical behaviour, including blasphemy, extortion, witchcraft, seduction, as well as being an observant Jew.

- The China Study makes several arguments, including that a plant-based diet 1) plays a critical role in determining how genes are expressed, either good or bad; 2) controls the negative effects of unhealthy chemicals, 3) can help resolve chronic diseases, and 4) will create health in all areas of our lives. The China Study also argues that there are no nutrients in animal proteins that are better than plant-based proteins.

- The China Study was a 20-year study that compared the mortality rates of meat eaters and plant eaters. They found that countries that ate more animal-based food were more likely to have higher death rates from "Western diseases," while countries that ate more plant food were healthier.

- The citrus soda 7-UP was created in 1929; "7" was selected because the original containers were 7 ounces. "UP" indicated the direction of the bubbles.

- The citrus soda 7-UP was created in 1929; "7" was selected because the original containers were 7 ounces. "UP" indicated the direction of the bubbles.

- The Code of Hammurabi (1800 B.C.) includes a law that punishes fraudulent wine sellers: They were to be drowned in a river

- The coffee industry employs 25 million people around the world.

- The combination of French fries and hamburgers is a continuation of the "meat and potatoes" mentality that has been the core of American food since the eighteenth century.

- The combination of soil type, climate, degree of slope, and exposure to the sun constitutes the terroir of a vineyard and what makes each vineyard and each wine unique.

- The consumption of natural vanilla causes the body to release catecholamine (including adrenalin) – for this reason it is considered to be mildly addictive.

- The country whose people eat the most chocolate is Switzerland, with 22 pounds eaten per person each year. Australia and Ireland follow with 20 pounds and 19 pounds per person, respectively. The United States comes in at 11th place, with approximately 12 pounds of chocolate eaten by each person every year.

- The creamy middle of a Twinkie is not cream at all but mostly Crisco, which is vegetable shortening.

- The digestive tract (alimentary canal) in humans includes the mouth, oesophagus, small intestine (duodenum, jejunum, illeum), and large intestine (caecum, colon, rectum, anus). The liver and pancreas are not part of the digestive tract but provide vital digestive secretions, such as bile and pancreatic juices.

- The Dust Bowl forced tens of thousands of farmers, known as Oakes, to leave their farms. The Dust Bowl exodus was the largest migration in American history.

- The Dutch were the first Europeans to enter the coffee trade. They imported coffee plants from the Malabar Coast of India to their colonies in what were then called the Dutch East Indies, or present-day Indonesia.

- The earliest recorded mention of a disease that can be recognized as diabetes is found in the Ebers papyrus (1500 B.C.), which includes directions for several mixtures that could "remove the urine, which runs too often."

- The Ebers papyrus (1350 B.C.) suggests placing drops of crushed and roasted ox liver in the eyes of people suffering from night blindness. While Egyptians most likely were not aware of vitamin A, liver does have high levels of the vitamin which help maintains normal vision in dim light.

- The English are sometimes called "limeys" because British sailors would eat limes to stave off scurvy. Limes were later replaced by lemons due to the lack of adequate vitamin C in lime juice.

- The English chocolate company Cadbury made the first chocolate bar in the world in 1842.

- The English word "wine" may be rooted in the Semitic yayin (lamentation and wailing). In Arabic, the word is wain, in Greek it is oinos, and in the Romance languages it is vin, vino, vina, vinho.

- The estimated annual medical cost of obesity in the U.S. was $147 billion in 2008. The medical costs for obese people were $1,429 higher than those of normal weight.

- The European Union declared that sparkling wine produced outside the French region of Champagne can no longer be labelled "champagne"

- The European Union, the U.S., Canada, Japan, and other countries require organic food producers to have a special certification based on government-defined standards to market food as organic.

- The fast food industry has dramatically affected how cattle and chickens are raised, slaughtered, and processed. It also encouraged consolidation in the meatpacking industry, such that there are now only 13 major meatpackers in America. McDonald's is the largest purchaser of beef and has great influence over meatpacking practices.

- The FDA is debating a proposal to allow candy makers to substitute vegetable oil for the traditional cacao butter.

- The Fertile Crescent is the site of the earliest planned sowing and harvesting of plants.

- The first chocolate chip cookie was invented in 1937 by Ruth Wakefield who ran the "Toll House Inn." The term "Toll House" is now legally a generic word for chocolate chip cookie. It is the most popular cookie worldwide and is the official cookie of Massachusetts.

- The first known illustration of wine drinking is found on a 5,000-year-old Sumerian panel known as the Standard of Ur.

- The first located printed reference to hamburgers appeared in the Los Angeles Times in 1894.

- The first machine-made chocolate was produced in Barcelona, Spain, in 1780.

- The first meal on the moon was roast turkey, eaten by Niel Armstrong and Buzz Aldrin.

- The first people to harvest chocolate were the Mokaya and other pre-Olmec peoples who lived in southeast Mexico around 1000 B.C. The word "chocolate" is derived from the Mayan word xocolatl, or "bitter water."

- The first product to have a bar code was Wrigley's gum.

- The first Renaissance figure to advocate vegetarianism was Leonardo da Vinci. However, other influential figures, such as Immanuel Kant and Rene Descartes, did not believe humans had any ethical obligations toward animals.

- The first Vegetarian Society was formed in England in 1847. The society's goal was to teach people that it is possible to be healthy without eating meat.

- The five countries with the highest percentage of diabetes are Nauru, United Arab Emirates, Saudi Arabia, Bahrain, and Kuwait.

- The flavour of zucchini is best when it is less than six inches long

- The four major biotech crops in 2012 were soybean, cotton, maize, and canola.

- The Germans invented Eiswein, or wine that is made from frozen grapes.

- The Greeks and Romans regulated nutrition on the theory of the four humours circulating throughout the body (warm, cold, moist, dry). Classical physicians tried to correct an excess of cold and moist "humours" by providing hot, dry foods and vice versa. For example, a woman's body was seen as wetter and colder than a man's and, therefore, she was to avoid food that would make her even colder and wetter, such as fish, eels, and meat from new-born animals.

- The heart rate of a person with anorexia might drop from a normal 60–100 beats per minute to lower than 60 beats a minute.

- The high water content in celery makes it ideal for vegetable juicing.

- The human body is equipped with 60,000 miles of blood vessels and wired with 100,000 miles of nerve fibres. Diabetes often blocks the cardiovascular system and deadens nerves, causing 80% of deaths among patients with diabetes.

- The human digestive system is home to between 10 and 100 trillion bacteria, at least 10 times the amount of cells in the body. Some scholars speculate that intestinal bacteria differ in lean and obese people.

- The ideal popping temperature for popcorn is 400-460° Fahrenheit. A kernel will pop, on average, when it reaches 347° Fahrenheit.

- The increase of junk food is directly associated with the increase in obesity, heart disease, high blood pressure, certain cancers, tooth decay, and other diseases.

- The Industrial Revolution led to faster and more efficient farming technology, which helped usher in the Second Agricultural Revolution from 1700 to 1900 in developed countries. Many less developed countries are still experiencing the Second Agricultural Revolution.

- The invention of the meat grinder in the mid nineteenth century gave rise to the hamburger. Currently, between 40,000 and 50,000 meatpackers, many of whom pack meat for fast food chains, are injured every year, making meatpacking one of the most dangerous jobs in the United States.

- The jambul fruit leaves and bark are used for controlling blood pressure and gingivitis.

- The juiciest, most delicious oranges in the world are grown in Florida.

- The largest and oldest chocolate company in the U.S. is Hershey's. Hershey's produces over one billion pounds of chocolate product annually.

- The largest cuckoo clock made of chocolate can be found in Germany.

- The leaves of celery are often bitter, so it is recommended to remove them before juicing.a

- The leaves of raspberry is used fresh or dried as herbal teas to regulate menstrual cycles

- The Lipton Tea Factory in Jebel Ali, Dubai, produces 5 billion tea bags a year.

- The liquid inside young coconuts can be used as substitute for blood plasma.

- The man who most profoundly affected the history of wine was the prophet Mohammed. Within ten years of his death in A.D. 632, wine was largely banned from Arabia and from every country that heeded him.

- The Mesopotamians built the first simple irrigation system around 7000 B.C. The earliest large-scale irrigation system was created around 4000 B.C. in southern Russia. This system had canals up to 10 feet across and more than a mile long.

- The most expensive chocolate in the world is the "Madeleine" and was created by Fritz Knipschildt of Knipschildt Chocolatier in Connecticut.

- The most expensive coffee in the world is Indonesia's Kopi Luwak or civet coffee. It is made from coffee beans that have been eaten, partially digested, and then excreted by a weasel-like animal called the Asian palm civet. These beans sell for more than $600 a pound, or $50 a cup.

- The most expensive tea in the world is a rare Chinese tea called Tieguanyin, which is around $1,500/lb. The tea is named after the Buddhist deity Guan Yin (Iron Goddess of Mercy). It is an oolong tea.

- The most expensive teapot in the world is a rare pair of "melon" teapots from 18th century China. They sold for $2.18 million. They had been owned by a Scottish collector who had them for 50 years but did not realize

- The most popular cookie in America is the chocolate chip cookie, which is attributed to Ruth Wakefield circa 1933.

- The name "diabetes" is attributed to the famed Greek physician Aretaeus of Cappadocia who practiced in the first century A.D. He believed that diabetes was caused by snakebite.

- The name pine-apple was the original name for a pine cone (grows on pine trees). Because the fruit pineapple looked like a huge pine cone, it too was called a pine-apple.

- The name Starbucks was inspired by a character in the novel Moby Dick. The owners almost named their coffee shop Pequod, another character in the novel.

- The National Association of Anorexia Nervosa and Associated Disorders reports that only 30–40% of anorexics ever fully recover.

- The number of animals killed for meat every hour in the U.S. is 500,000.

- The number of reported cases of anorexia in young women between 15 and 19 has risen each decade since 1930.

- The number of reported cases of bulimia in females ages 10-39 tripled between 1988 and 1993.

- The oldest ear of popcorn was found in a bat cave in Mexico in 1948. It is believed to be over 5,000 years old.

- The two places in North America where coffee is grown are in Hawaii and Puerto Rico.

- The only vegetables with all eight types of essential amino acids in sufficient amounts are lupin beans, soy, hempseed, chia seed, amaranth, buckwheat, and quinoa. However, the essential amino acids can be achieved by eating other vegetables if they are in a variety.

- The organic food movement began in the 1940s in response to the Green Revolution. The Green Revolution marked a significant increase in food production due to the introduction of high-yield varieties, the use of pesticides, and better management techniques.

- The peanut is actually a legume, not a nut (which is why they are often roasted).

- The phrase "buy the farm" is WWII slang meaning to die or get killed.

- The phrase "fetch the farm" is prisoner slang from at least 1879 for "get sent to the infirmary," where there is a better diet and not as much hard labour.

- The physician to Queen Victoria, Sir William Gull (1816-1890), was the first to coin the term anorexia nervosa in his text Anorexia Hysterica. His work helped move the study of anorexia into the field of psychiatry.

- The popularization of drive-thru restaurants has led to the development of increasingly sophisticated cup holders in cars

- The popularization of the automobile resulted in "flashier" fast food restaurant architecture to catch the attention of drivers. This lasted until the 1970s when communities began to complain about the exaggerated buildings.

- The popularization of the drive-thru led car manufacturers in the 1990s to install cup holders in the dashboards. As fast food drinks became larger, so did the cup holders.

- The prohibitionists, or the "drys," in the early twentieth century fought to remove any mention of wine from school and college texts, including Greek and Roman literature. They also sought to remove medicinal wines from the United States Pharmacopoeia and to prove that Biblical praises of wine were for unfermented grape juice.

- The rates of obesity in America's children and youth have almost tripled in the last quarter century, and children are the fastest growing segment of the obese population in the U.S. Today's children consume multiple types of media and spend more time in front of computers, TV, and game screens than any other activity in their lives except sleeping.

- The reason fewer boys develop eating disorders may be that they are older when they reach puberty and may be more emotionally prepared to deal with their changing bodies. Additionally, boys tend to be less critical of their bodies than girls.

- The rise in the fast food industry has been linked to rising cases of obesity. The CDC estimates that 248,000 Americans die prematurely due to obesity and considers obesity as the number two cause of preventable death in the US (the #1 cause is smoking).

- The Ritz Carlton of Hong Kong has the world's most expensive High Tea meal, at a price of $8,888 per couple.

- The scientific name for popcorn is Zea Mays Everta. It is a type of maize, a member of the Maydeae tribe in the large, natural order of grasses called the Graminae.

- The smell of burning wood is the most recognizable odour in America. The smell of coffee is the second.

- The smell of young wine is called an "aroma" while a more mature wine offers a more subtle "bouquet."

- The softer the texture of a fruit or vegetable, the thicker the juice produced. Apricots, peaches, pears, melons, and strawberries are soft-textured fruits, so their juice is very thick. Many raw foodists combine these juices with thinner juices, such as carrot or apple.

- The soluble fibre in oatmeal helps control blood glucose levels

- The song "I'm a Little Teapot, Short and Stout" was written in 1939 by Tin Pan Ally songwriters Clarence Kelley and George Harry Sanders.

- The spread of chocolate from Spain throughout Europe began in the sixteenth century with the expulsion of Jews from Spain and Portugal during the Inquisition. Some Jews who left Spain brought with them Spain's secrets of processing chocolate.

- The standard wine container of the ancient world was the amphora (something which can be carried by two), a clay vase with two handles. It was invented by the Canaanites, who introduced it into Egypt before the fifteenth century B.C. Their forebears, the Phoenicians, spread its use throughout the Mediterranean.

- The study of obesity is known as bariatric, from the Greek root bar- or "weight" (as in barometer), -iatr or "treatment" (as in pediatrics), and -ic or"pertaining to." The term was created around 1965. As obesity has become a major health problem in the United States, bariatrics has become a separate medical and surgical specialtyn.

- The substance in wine that tingles the gums is tannin (related to the word "tan"), which is derived from the skins, pips, and stalks of grapes. It is usually found only in red wine and is an excellent antioxidant. Visually, it is the sediment found at the bottom of the bottle.

- The tallest, biggest trees or bushes do not always yield the most fruit. Controlling the height of plants helps produce more fruit in less space. Farmers may also change a tree's shape by cutting branches or forcing branches to grow in a certain direction. The shape of the tree affects its lifespan and the size of its fruit.

- The tannic acid in black tea is said to help remove warts.

- The tannins found in green tea have been found to help stop bleeding by coagulating the blood.

- The term "cholesterol" is from the Greek khole or "bile" (as in "cholera") + sterops or "solid, stiff" (as in "sterility").

- The term "herbal tea" means that the tea has been infused with herbs or fruit that was not part of the tea plant. Herbal tea includes rosehip and chamomile teas.

- The term "junk food" was initially used in the 1960s but was popularized during the following decade when the song "Junk Food Junkie" reached the top of the charts in 1976.

- The term "vitamin" was coined by Polish-American chemist Casimir Funk and is derived from vital (necessary for life) and amine (a compound containing nitrogen and hydrogen). It was later discovered that not all vitamins are amines. Vitamins were discovered one at a time from 1900-1950. Many vitamins cannot be synthesized by the body in adequate amounts and must be obtained from the diet.

- The terroir of wine differentiates and adds value to wine

- The Third Agricultural Revolution, or the Green Revolution, corresponds in the late 20th century with the exponential population growth occurring around the world. It includes biotechnology, genetic engineering, chemical fertilizers, and mass production of agricultural goods.

- The Tootsie Roll is named after its creator Leo Hirshfield's daughter Clara, whose nickname was Tootsie. It was the first penny candy that was individually wrapped. During WWII, Tootsie Rolls were placed in soldiers' ration kits because they could survive various weather conditions.

- The total production of excrement by the U.S. population is 12,000 pounds per second. The total production of excrement by U.S. livestock is 250,000 pounds per second, which would be greatly reduced if humans ate a more plant-based diet and had little or no need for domesticated livestock. Less livestock would also greatly reduce Earth's trapped greenhouse gases.

- The Turks call their coffee houses "schools for the wise."

- The Twinkie derived its name after bakery manager Jimmy Dewar saw an advertisement for the "Twinkle Toe Shoe Company" on a trip to St. Louis in the 1920s. They became the bestselling snack cake in the United States after WWII and have appeared in many movies such as Ghostbusters (1984), Grease (1978), and Sleepless in Seattle (1993).

- The U.S. economy loses an estimated $270 billion annually in health care costs and loss of productivity associated with obesity and overweight workers. Obesity also resulted in 39 million lost workdays.

- The U.S. Human Genome Project linked a pregnant woman's cholesterol deficiency to a defect in the fetal brain called HPE (the failure of the brain to divide normally into two halves). Ninety-nine percent of embryos with HPE are spontaneously aborted. Those which do live usually die within the first year of life and experience severe mental retardation. Consequently, pregnant women are often advised not to take cholesterol-lowering drugs.

- The United States exported $136 billion in farm goods in 2011, with a $37 billion trade surplus.

- The United States invented both the tea bag and iced tea in 1904. Many tea lovers consider the tea bag as one of the worst inventions of the 20th century. Tea brewed with loose tea is generally considered to be richer than tea made from bags.

- The United States, Brazil, Argentina, Canada, and India plant most of the GMO cropland. More than 152 million of the world's 170 million GMO hectares are found in these five countries.

- The USDA National Organic Standards prohibit the use of genetically modified organisms (GMOs) in products that are labelled "100% organic." However, the contamination of the crops may cause some organic food to contain some GMO traces.

- The vegetarian movement has been influenced by ancient ethics of abstinence, early medical science that noted similarities between humans and animals, and Indian philosophy that promotes kindness to animals.

- The Vikings called America Vinland ("wine-land" or "pasture-land") for the profusion of native grape vines they found there around A.D. 1000.

- The vintage year isn't necessarily the year wine is bottled, because some wines may not be bottled the same year the grapes are picked. Typically, a vintage wine is a product of a single year's harvest. A non-vintage wine is a blend of wines from two or more years.

- The word "champagne" is named after a province in France, meaning "open country. Due to the Protected Designation of Origin (PDO) law in Europe, sparkling wine made outside the Champagne region of France can no longer be called "champagne."

- The word "coffee" is from the Arabic qahwah, which is thought to have meant "wine." The Turkish word for coffee, kahve, is derived from the Arabic word and is related to the word café. Other scholars believe the word is from Kaffa, a region in Ethiopia where coffee is thought to have originated.

- The word "diabetes" is Greek for "siphon," which refers to the copious urine of uncontrolled diabetes. "Mellitus" is Latin for "honey" or "sweet," a name added when physicians discovered that the urine from people with diabetes is sweet with glucose.

- The word "farm" is from the Old French ferme, meaning to "rent, lease," and the Latin firmare, "to fix, settle, confirm, strengthen."

- The word "health" comes from the Anglo-Saxon term hal meaning "wholeness."

- The word "vegan" is derived from the word "vegetarian." It was first used in 1944 when Elsie Shrigley and Donald Watson thought that the word "vegetarian" included too many types of animal by-products and did not encompass a completely plant-based diet.

- The World Health Organization (WHO) reports that diabetes has reached epidemic proportions and expects that 80% of all new cases of diabetes will appear in developing countries by 2025.

- The world population will jump from 7 billion to 9 billion by 2050. Farmers will need to double food production by then to keep pace.

- The world's first coffee house opened in 1475 in Constantinople (modern-day Istanbul).

- The world's largest popcorn ball was 12 feet in diameter and weighed 5,000 pounds. It required 2,000 pounds of corn, 40,000 pounds of sugar, 280 gallons of corn syrup, and 400 gallons of water.

- The world's oldest bottle of wine dates back to A.D. 325 and was found near the town of Speyer, Germany, inside one of two Roman sarcophaguses. It is on display at the town's Historisches Museum der Pfalz.

- The world's oldest known popper, a shallow vessel with a handle and hole on top was designed around A.D. 300. The first popcorn machine made its debut 1,500 years later at the 1893 World's Fair (Columbian Exposition) in Chicago.

- The world's largest wine cask is in Heidelberg, Germany.

- The world's oldest piece of chewing gums is 9000 years old.

- The worst place to store wine is usually in the kitchen because it is typically too warm to store wine safely. Refrigerators are not satisfactory for storing wine either. Even at their warmest setting, they're too cold.

- There are 18 different animal shapes in the Animal Crackers cookie zoo!

- There are 6 basic categories of tea: 1) white, 2) yellow, 3) green, 4) oolong, 5) black, 6) and post-fermented.

- There are about 1 million people in the United States with Type 1 diabetes, but only 2,000 donor pancreases are available each year for transplants.

- There are about 1,600 popcorn kernels in 1 cup.

- There are actually zero cacao solids in white chocolate.

- There are approximately 60 nutrients which are placed in six major categories: proteins, carbohydrates, fats, vitamins, minerals, and water.

- There are around 2.2 million farms in the United States.

- There are enough calories in 217 Big Macs to drive a small car for 88 miles. There are enough calories in 1 piece of cheesecake to light a 60-watt bulb for 1½ hours.

- There are more than 300,000 fast food restaurants in the U.S. alone.

- There are more than 7,000 varieties of apples grown in the world.

- There are over 20 chemicals commonly used in the growing and processing of organic crops that are approved by the U.S. Organic Standards. The actual use of pesticides used by organic farms is not recorded by the government. Many natural pesticides have been found to have dangerous health risks.

- There are over 200 different known species of raspberries but only 2 species are grown on a large scale.

- There are over 500 different types of bananas. That means if you ate a different kind of banana every day, it would take almost a year and a half to eat every one!

- There are over 7000 different types of apples grown all over the world.

- There are seven varieties of avocados grown commercially in Texas, but the Hass is the most popular.

- There are several types of vegetarians. The strictest type is vegans. Vegans avoid not only meat but also all animal products. There is a debate within the vegan community about whether honey is appropriate for a vegan diet. For example, the Vegan Society and the American Vegan Society do not consider honey appropriate because it comes from an animal.

- There are six major maize types: pod corn, sweet corn, flour corn, dent corn, flint corn, and popcorn. Popcorn kernels come in three shapes: rice, pearl, and South American. Most commercial popcorn is the pearl type. The major trait shared by all types of popcorn kernels is their ability to explode and create a flake when kernels are exposed to heat.

- There are two basic juicers available on the market: centrifugal juice extractors and cold press juicers (a.k.a. masticating juicers). Specialists suggest buying a centrifugal juicer if you a) want to use the juice mostly for cooking, baking, or other processes where the juice will eventually be exposed to heat, b) don't mind if it is less efficient at extracting all the nutrients, and c) are trying to save cash. A cold press juicer is more helpful if you a) are interested in cleansing, making nut milks and green juices, and fresher juices, b) want to pack as many nutrients into your body as possible, and c) can afford a more expensive juicer.

- There are two different words for tea: te-derived (Min, a historical Chinese language) and cha-derived (Cantonese and Mandarin). The word a specific country uses for tea reveals where the country first acquired its tea.

- There are two main species of the coffee plant used to commercially produce coffee: 1) Coffee arabica, which originated in the Middle East, and 2) Coffea Robusta, which originated in the Congo. Arabica trees produce the best quality coffee and are the most widely cultivated (3/4 of the world's coffee), while Robusta beans are hardier, contain 40-50% more caffeine, and are used in many instant coffees.

- There is a right and wrong way to hold a wine glass. Wine glasses should always be held by the stem and not the bowl because the heat of the hand will raise the temperature of the wine.

- There is an estimated 1,500 different types of tea.

- There is increasing scientific evidence that moderate, regular wine drinking can reduce the risk of heart disease, Alzheimer's disease, stroke, and gum disease.

- There were 6.4 million visits to doctors' offices that involved a cholesterol test. That is 7.1% of all visits.

- They also contain aflatoxin, a carcinogenic, which may explain why peanut farmers have been found

- Those with diabetes are more likely to develop carpal tunnel syndrome and tarsal tunnel syndrome.

- Those with diabetes, particularly adolescent girls with Type 1 diabetes, may be at increased risk of developing eating disorders. Some adolescent girls purposely withhold their insulin to lose weight.

- Though coffee was discovered in Ethiopia around A.D. 850, it wasn't until it spread to Mocha, Yemen, in around 1100 that it became firmly established as a popular drink. From Mocha (from which Mocha coffee derives its name), beans were shipped to India, Java, and eventually Europe in 1515. By 1675, England had more than 3,000 coffee houses.

- Though heart disease has dropped among non-diabetic women by 27%, it has actually increased by 23% for women with diabetes.

- Though the Eastern world has been using tea for more than 4,500, tea was introduced to the West only 400 years ago.

- Three studies in 2011 showed that pregnant women exposed to higher amounts of organophosphate pesticides, which are used in conventional farming, ended up having children with lower IQs than those of their peers.

- Thrifty" genes, or genes that helped convert excess calories into fat that provided energy during lean times in the past, are now contributing to obesity. Approximately 90% of those of African descent have "thrifty" genes, around 50% of Asians have them, and about 20–35% of Europeans have them.

- Thucydides wrote that the people of the Mediterranean began to "emerge from barbarism when they learned to cultivate the oil and the vine."

- Tips coffee mug Coffee is the world's second most traded commodity .More than 500 billion cups of coffee are consumed each year, making coffee the world's most popular beverage. It is also the world's most traded commodity, after crude oil.

- To increase the protein in peanut butter (peanuts have about the same amount of protein as soy), Brewer's yeast can be mixed in. This is especially useful for vegetarian

- To keep salaries low, McDonald's and other fast food chains have intentionally engaged in anti-union activities.

- To make juice clear, filter juice through layers of cheesecloth or a nut milk bag. This will also remove any foam that forms during juicing. You may also strain the juice through a fine mesh strainer to reduce pulp and foam.

- To make juice more balanced with protein, raw foodists suggest adding almond milk, Greek yogurt, flaxseed, or peanut butter.

- To obtain the maximum nutritional benefits, onions should be eaten raw or lightly steamed

- To produce enough beans to make one cup of coffee requires 37 gallons of water. By comparison, an apple takes 19 gallons, a banana 27, and a pair of leather shoes 4,400 gallons.

- To stop mindless eating, experts recommend eating foods low in calories and high in fibre and water, using smaller plates and serving utensils, being aware of the "clean plate mentality," avoiding all-you-can-eat restaurants and buffets, and not doing other activities while eating, such as watching T.V.

- Today the United States has a $23 billion candy market. Candy sales have continued to increase despite concerns with junk food and obesity.

- Today, Americans consume approximately 70 million "tater tots" a year. They were created to utilize potato shreds left over from french fry production. The film Napoleon Dynamite (2004) popularized them even more. To burn off one serving (3 oz) of tater tots would take about 67 minutes of walking

- Today, Americans consume approximately 70 million "tator tots" a year. The film Napoleon Dynamite (2004) popularized them even more

- Today, Coca-Cola and PepsiCo products are sold in every country in the world, except North Korea.

- Today's farmers grow more than "food, feed, and fibre"—they also grow crops that are processed into fuel. For example, corn can be made into ethanol and soybean oil can be made into diesel fuel.

- Tomatoes are a fruit not a vegetable. Tomatoes are the most popular fruits in the world.

- Tomatoes are an excellent source of vitamin C (the vitamin C is most concentrated in the

- Tomatoes are rich in lycopene, flavonoids and other phytochemicals with ant carcinogenic properties

- Total cholesterol levels (the combination of "good" HDL cholesterol and "bad" LDL cholesterol) that are more than 200 mg/dL are considered to be unhealthy. Nearly half of all American adults have a cholesterol level at or more than 200 mg/dL.

- Total global cropland amounts to roughly 1.5 billion hectares. Genetically modified organisms (GMOs) make up more than 11% of all cropland in the world.

- Tractors were invented in the 1880s to pull ploughs through fields. By the 1920s the all purpose, modern tractor had been developed. With different attachments, tractors can be used for ploughing, planting, cultivating, mowing, harvesting, and moving soil and heavy equipment.

- Traditionally, wine was never stored standing up. Keeping the wine on its side kept the wine in contact with the cork, thereby preventing the cork from drying, shrinking, and letting in air. However, wine can be stored vertically if the bottle has an artificial cork.

- Tumours and lesions in the brain have been associated with the development of abnormal eating patterns and symptoms of eating disorders.

- Twelve million men (11.2% of all men 20 years and older) and 11.5 million women (10.2% of all women 20 years and older) have diabetes in the U.S.

- Two fast food chains claim to have opened the first drive-ins: Pig Stand, which opened in 1921 in Texas, and A&W Root Beer, which launched in California in 1919.

- Two tablespoons of un-popped kernels produce a quart of popcorn for about 25 cents.

- Two-thirds of Americans are overweight. Weight gained after one's early twenties is linked to higher chances of suffering from heart disease, cancer, infertility, gallstones, asthma, and even snoring.

- Two-thirds of the world's eggplant is grown in New Jersey.

"Our bodies are our gardens – our wills are our gardeners."

~William Shakespeare

CHAPTER 20

U- LIFESTYLE

- U.S. chocolate manufacturers use about 3.5 million pounds of whole milk every day to make milk chocolate.

- U.S. dairy farmers receive less than $1.32 per gallon of milk they produce. The average retail price of milk $2.76. The average cow produces 7 gallons of milk a day, 2,100 pounds of milk a month, and 46,000 glasses of milk a year. There are 350 squirts in a gallon of milk.

- Unplanned pregnancies are four times higher among singe obese women than normal-weight women, even though obese women were 30% less likely to have had a sexual partner in the past year.

- Un-popped popcorn kernels are called "spinsters" or "old maids." Quality popcorn should produce 98% popped kernels with under 2% being spinsters

- Un-popped popcorn makes up about 90% of sales for home consumption.

- Un-popped popcorn should not be stored in the refrigerator. The refrigerator will dry out the moisture in the kernels. Without the moisture, popcorn will not pop. The ideal place to store popcorn is in a cool, dry cupboard.

"It's bizarre that the produce manager is more important to my children's health than the pediatrician."

~Meryl Streep

CHAPTER 21

V- LIFESTYLE

- Vegan diet A variety of plant sources can provide a vegetarian/vegan diet with enough protein Vegetarians have only slightly lower protein intake than those with a meat diet. Various studies around the world confirm that vegetarian diets provide enough protein if they include a variety of plant sources.

- Vegetarianism has roots in ancient India. In fact, currently 70% of the world's vegetarians are Indians and there are more vegetarians in India than in any other country in the world.

- Vegetarianism is based in the ancient Indian and Greek philosophies. India, vegetarianism was based on the philosophy of ahimsa or nonviolence toward animals. For the Hellenes and Egyptians, it had ritual or medical purposes. After Rome became Christianized, vegetarianism largely disappeared from Europe. It remerged in the Renaissance.

- Vegetarianism is still required for yogis in Hatha Yoga and Bhakti Yoga. Eating meat is said to lead to ignorance, sloth, and an undesirable mental state known as tamas. A vegetarian diet, on the other hand, leads to sattvic qualities that are associated with spiritual progress.

- Vegetarians can be deficient in Vitamin B12, which only comes from animal sources (though it can also be in fortified yeast extract products). Research suggests that a Vitamin B12 deficiency may be tied to the weakening of bones.

- Vegetarians such as the Manicheans and Cathars were considered heretics and persecuted during the medieval Inquisition.

- Vending machines were developed in the United Kingdom in the 1880s and were used to sell gum at train stations in New York. By 1926, there was one vending machine for every 100 people in America.

- Vitamin B12 deficiency can lead to anaemia, neural disorders, and psychotic behaviour. Women who are planning to get pregnant are encouraged to have healthy levels of Vitamin B12 to prevent potential birth defects.

- Vitamin D is unusual because it is the only vitamin that can be synthesized in the body. Sunlight is the main source of Vitamin D, though sunscreen lotions with high SPF can prevent vitamin D formation. Vitamin D is also the only vitamin that is a hormone.

- Vitamins are grouped according to their solubility in either fat or water. Vitamins A, D, E, and K are fat soluble, meaning they need fat to be absorbed into the body and can be stored in the body. Vitamin B complexes and Vitamin C are water soluble and, because they cannot be stored in the body, they must be replaced every day.

"By cleansing your body on a regular basis and eliminating as many toxins as possible from your environment, your body can begin to heal itself, prevent disease, and become stronger and more resilient than you ever dreamed possible!"

~Dr. Edward Group III

CHAPTER 22

W- LIFESTYLE

- Washing produce does not completely remove pesticides

- Water accounts for 55-70% of our body weight, and typically a minimum of six to eight glasses of water is needed to keep the body performing at optimal levels (the amount of water needed differs according to an individual's health, physical activity, environment, etc). A 20% loss of fluid from the body is usually fatal. Conversely, drinking too much water can also be fatal.

- Weight loss in anorexics is most obvious in the arms and legs. The loss of subcutaneous fat (fat directly under the skin layers) makes the shape of the bones very easy to see.

- Well known people with diabetes include Mary Tyler Moore, Jerry Mathers (Leave it to Beaver), and Jerry Garcia of The Grateful Dead. The late Carroll O'Conner from the TV show All in the Family had diabetes and had his toe amputated in 2000.

- Western diets often include snacking on junk food filled with sugar. Consequently, insulin remains high throughout the day, which can cause metabolic problems including type 2 diabetes.

- When an egg floats in water, it is "off" and should not be eaten.

- When buying peanut butter, only buy organic varieties.

- When choosing raw fruits and veggies to juice, terms such as "pasteurized" and "hydrogenated" indicate that the food has been heated above the 118° threshold, which make them cooked—not raw—foods.

- When English Buccaneers overran a Spanish ship loaded with cacao beans, they set it on fire, thinking the beans were sheep dung.

- When explorer Felix de Azara visited Paraguay in the 18th century, he noted that the people would place kernels on a tassel and then when it was boiled in fat or oil, the grains would burst. Women would adorn their hair at night with the popcorn.

- When France refused to join the American-led coalition against Iraq, some Republicans argued that the name French fries be changed to "liberty fries."

- When honey is swallowed, it enters the blood stream within a period of 20 minutes.

- When it was revealed in 1990 that McDonald's used beef tallow to flavour its French fries, Hindu vegetarian customers in Mumbai (formerly Bombay), India, ransacked a McDonald's restaurant and smeared cow dung on a statue of Ronald MacDonald.

- When Khair Bey, the governor of Mecca, banned coffee in 1511 because he feared it might encourage resistance to his rule, the sultan executed him on the grounds that coffee was actually "blessed."

- When McDonald's opened an outlet in Kuwait shortly after the end of the Gulf War, the line of cars waiting to eat there was seven miles long.

- When organic food travels long distances to market (food miles), it creates pollution that may offset any positive environmental effects of organic farming. However, buying local food, which may or may not be grown organically, helps reduce the environmental costs associated with food miles.

- When tasting wine, hold the wine in the mouth for a moment or two and then either swallow it or, preferably, spit it out, usually into a spittoon. A really good wine will have a long aftertaste, while an inferior wine will have a short aftertaste.

- When tea is being poured in China, guests tap two or three fingers on the table three times to show gratitude to the server.

- When televisions became popular in the early 1950s, popcorn sales decreased because people stayed home to watch movies rather than go to a theatre. However, when popcorn was more readily available at home, popcorn again became popular.

- When the first coffeehouse opened in England in 1652, women were prohibited from entering, other than to serve men.

- When Tutankhamen's tomb was opened in 1922, the wine jars buried with him were labelled with the year, the name of the winemaker, and comments such as "very good wine." The labels were so specific that they could actually meet modern wine label laws of several countries.

- When wine and food are paired together, they have "synergy" or a third flavor beyond what either the food or drink offers alone.

- While 1,120 litres of water go into producing a single litre of coffee, only 120 litres go into making the same amount of tea. In fact, to produce one litre of tea takes less water than producing wine, apple juice, orange juice, or beer.

- While all pits, such as plum pits and peach pits, should be removed before juicing, the seeds of citrus fruits, grapes, papaya, and melons may be put through the juicer.

- While eating a plant-based diet is linked to lower risk of heart disease and cancer, there is not significant research linking the health benefits to juicing specifically.

- While fans of juicing claim that juicing is better than eating whole fruits and veggies because the body does not have to work to process fibre, most people do not receive the recommended amount of fibre per day anyway.

- While Hispanics have a higher rate of Type 2 diabetes than non-Hispanic whites, they typically live longer than non-Hispanic whites on kidney dialysis.

- While Hitler wasn't willing to institute the policy during World War II, he did believe that vegetarianism could be key to Germany's military success. He claimed that Caesar's soldiers lived entirely on vegetables and the Vikings wouldn't have been able to undertake their expeditions if they depended on a meat diet.

- While in older times it was customary to pour the milk first into a tea cup as a way to protect the surface of the china, tea connoisseurs say that is not necessary now. Instead it is better to pour the milk in after the tea because it is easier to judge how much is needed.

- While it is a popular story, there is no evidence that Native Americans brought the Pilgrims popcorn at the Thanksgiving dinner. While Native Americans in South America, Central America, and the south-western region of the U.S ate popcorn, there is no evidence that Native Americans in Massachusetts or Virginia did.

- While juice can provide the same calcium as milk, milk may be more satisfying than raw juice because milk has more protein. Some juices also have more calories than milk.

- While liver is an iron-rich food, it is also high in cholesterol. In fact, the most concentrated levels of cholesterol in animal meats are found in organ meats like the liver. Three ounces of cooked liver contains 331 mg. of cholesterol.

- While mustard greens sold in the United States are relatively mild in flavour, some mustard green varieties, especially those in Asia, can be as hot as a jalapeno pepper depending on their mustard oil content

- While organic farmers say that they do not routinely treat their animals with antibiotics, a 2006 study found that a quarter of organic pigs had pneumonia compared to 4% of conventionally raised pigs and their piglets died twice as often.

- While organic food contains less pesticide residue, most conventional produce also has levels of residue below the threshold deemed unsafe.

- While organic potatoes use less energy in terms of fertilizer production, they need more fossil fuel for ploughing.

- While other businesses failed during the Great Depression, the popcorn business thrived. Popcorn sold at around 5 to 10 cents a bag, making it one of the more affordable (and possibly lifesaving) treats for poor families.

- While oysters and chocolate are well-known aphrodisiacs, juiced celery and watermelon can also boost sex drive. For example, celery increases male pheromones and watermelon helps relax blood vessels that increase the libido. Avocados contain a vitamin B, which is said to boost male hormone production.

- While raw food dieticians recommend giving up coffee, if a person must drink it, they suggest drinking it at least 30 minutes before or after drinking a fruit or vegetable juice. Coffee and caffeine are highly acidic, dehydrating, and taxing to the body.

- While seafood, such as fish, can be healthy, other types of seafood can have high levels of cholesterol. Just 3 oz. of lobster, for example, contains 61 mg. of cholesterol—before it is dipped in butter.

- While there may not be a significant difference nutritionally between organic and conventional foods, detectable pesticide residues were found in only 7% of organic product samples compared to 38% of conventional produce samples.

- While vegetarian diets tend to be lower in calories and higher in fibre (which makes a person feel more full), some vegetarian diets can cause higher caloric intake than a meat diet if they include a lot of cheese and nuts.

- While washing fruits and vegetables does reduce pesticide residue, some pesticides are absorbed internally in the plant and cannot be washed off. Others are formulated to bind to the surface of the crop and do not easily wash off. Peeling reduces exposure, but valuable nutrients are lost with the peel.

- While wine offers certain medical benefits, it may slightly increase the risk of contracting certain kinds of cancer of the digestive tract, particularly the oesophagus. There is also a slightly increased risk of breast cancer.

- White Castle, started by J. Walter Anderson and Edgar Waldo "Billy" Ingram, is considered to be the first fast food restaurant. Its major product was a hamburger, which had been sold as sandwiches by street vendors since the 1890s.

- White children have a greater risk of developing Type 1 diabetes than children of other races, though the incidence of the disease varies greatly from country to country. Risk factors include being ill in early infancy, having an older mother, having a mother with Type 1 diabetes, having a mother who had preeclampsia during pregnancy, and having a high birth weight.

- White tea is the least processed type of tea. The most "fussy" type of tea is oolong tea.

- Whole Foods is the largest retail giant in the natural food sector in the U.S with 360 stores in 40 U.S. states, Canada, and Britain. Its sales for fiscal 2012 year reached $11.7 billion.

- Whole Foods was started at the corner of 8th and Rio Grande in Austin, TX, in 1978 by self-described "free market" libertarian and now CEO, John Mackey. Originally called "Safer Way," it grew throughout the 1990s by absorbing its competitors: Bread & Circus, Fresh Fields, Merchant of Vino, Mrs. Gooch's, Bread of Life, and Wellspring Markets. Today, its only contenders are Wild Oats and Trader Joe's.

- William Cullen (1710-1790), a professor of chemistry and medicine in Scotland, is responsible for adding the term "mellitus" ("sweet" or "honey-like") to the word diabetes.

- Wine facilitated contacts between ancient cultures, providing the motive and means of trade. For example, the Greeks traded wine for precious metals, and the Romans traded wine for slaves.

- Wine for Orthodox Jews must be kosher, meaning it must not be touched at any point in its process (from picking of the grapes to bottling it) by either a "Gentile" or non-observant Jew and it must contain only kosher ingredients.

- Wine grapes rank number one among the world's fruit crops in terms of acres planted.

- Wine has a more concentrated effect on women than on men

- Wine often creates an exciting "synergy" with food

- Wine testers swirl their glass to encourage the wine to release all of its powerful aromas. Most don't fill the glass more than a third full in order to allow aromas to collect and to not spill it during a swirl.

- Winemaking is a significant theme in one of the oldest literary works known, the Epic of Gilgamesh. The divinity in charge of the wine was the goddess Siduri, whose depiction suggests a symbolic association between wine and fertility.

- Wineskins were a common way to transport wine in the ancient world. Animal skins (usually pig) were cleaned and tanned and turned inside out so that the hairy side was in contact with the wine.

- With age, red wines tend to lose colour and will eventually end up a sort of brick red. On the other hand, white wines gain colour, becoming golden and eventually brown-yellow.

- With more than four billion coffee trees, Brazil is the world's leading producer of coffee. In fact, Brazil produces around one third of the world's coffee today. Vietnam, Indonesia, Colombia, and India round out the top five coffee-producing countries.

- woman breast feeding The cholesterol in breast milk helps build nerve tissue in an infant's growing brain

- Women are more susceptible to the effects of wine than men partly because they have less of an enzyme in the lining of the stomach that is needed to metabolize alcohol efficiently.

- Women who are obese as they near retirement age are more likely to become disabled in their remaining years, with their risk of disability rising with their level of obesity. Nearly one third of U.S. women 75 years and older are obese.

- Women with college degrees are less likely to be obese compared with less educated women. However, there is no significant relationship between education and obesity among men.

- Women with diabetes are more likely to develop vaginal infections than are non-diabetics because of their elevated glucose levels.

- Women with post-traumatic stress disorder are more likely to be overweight or obese than women without the condition. One in nine women will have post-traumatic stress disorder (PTSD) at some point in her life, which is twice as often as men.

- Worldwide, consumers spend more than $7 billion a year on chocolate. Annual per capita consumption of chocolate is 12 pounds per person.

"It is health that is the

real wealth and not pieces

of gold and silver,"

Mahatma Gandhi.

CHAPTER 23

Y-Z- LIFESTYLE

- Yellow fruits help keep you from getting sick.

- You can make furniture with Pear wood (it's hard).

- You can make nitro-glycerine by peanut oil, which is a main part of dynamite.

- You can speed up the ripening of a pineapple by standing it upside down (on the leafy end).

- You'll eat about 35,000 cookies in a lifetime!

- Young women who eat a junk food diet are at a higher risk for developing Polycystic Ovarian Syndrome (PCOS).

- Your stomach has to produce a new layer of mucus every two weeks otherwise it will digest itself

- Zucchini and other summer squash varieties contain vitamins A and C

- Zucchinis can grow as large as baseball bats but have little flavour when they reach this size

www.ingramcontent.com/pod-product-compliance
Lightning Source LLC
Chambersburg PA
CBHW020423290526
45785CB00002B/699